Topics in Anaesthesia and Critical Care

H.K.F. VAN SAENE, L. SILVESTRI, M.A. DE LA CAL (EDS)
Infection Control in the Intensive Care Unit
1998, 380 pp, ISBN 3-540-75043-6

J. MILIC-EMILI (ED)
Applied Physiology in Respiratory Mechanics
1998, 246 pp, ISBN 3-540-75041-X

G. GUARNIERI, F. ISCRA (EDS)
Metabolism and Artificial Nutrition in the Critically Ill
1999, 130 pp, ISBN 88-470-0042-4

J. MILIC-EMILI, U. LUCANGELO, A. PESENTI, W.A. ZIN (EDS)
Basics of Respiratory Mechanism and Artificial Ventilation
1999, 268 pp, ISBN 88-470-0046-7

M. TIENGO, V.A. PALADINI, N. RAWAL (EDS)
Regional Anaesthesia, Analgesia and Pain Management
1999, 362 pp, ISBN 88-470-0044-0

I. SALVO, D. VIDYASAGAR (EDS)
Anaesthesia and Intensive Care in Neonates and Children
1999, 324 pp, ISBN 88-470-0043-2

G. BERLOT, H. DELOOZ, A. GULLO (EDS)
Trauma Operative Procedures
1999, 210 pp, ISBN 88-470-0045-9

G.L. ATLEE, J.-L. VINCENT (EDS)
Critical Care Cardiology in the Perioperative Period
2000, 214 pp, ISBN 88-470-0133-1

M.A. TIENGO (ED)
Neuroscience: Focus on Acute and Chronic Pain
2000, 214 pp, ISBN 88-470-0134-X

Anestesia e Medicina Critica

G. SLAVICH (ED)
Elettrocardiografia Clinica
1997, 328 pp, ISBN 3-540-75050-9

G.L. ALATI, B. ALLARIA, G. BERLOT, A. GULLO, A. LUZZANI,
G. MARTINELLI, L. TORELLI (EDS)
Anestesia e Malattie Concomitanti - Fisiopatologia e clinica del
periodo perioperatorio
1997, 382 pp, ISBN 3-540-75048-7

B. ALLARIA, M.V. BALDASSARE, A. GULLO, A. LUZZANI,
G. MANANI, G. MARTINELLI, A. PASETTO, L. TORELLI (EDS)
Farmacologia Generale e Speciale in Anestesiologia Clinica
1997, 312 pp, ISBN 88-470-0001-7

A. GULLO (ED)
Anestesia Clinica
1998, 506 pp, ISBN 88-470-0038-6

A. GULLO, L. GATTINONI
Medicina Intensiva e Perioperatoria
2000, 863 pp, ISBN 88-470-0135-8

Neuroscience: Focus on Acute and Chronic Pain

Springer

Milano
Berlin
Heidelberg
New York
Barcelona
Hong Kong
London
Paris
Singapore
Tokyo

M.A. Tiengo (Ed)

Neuroscience: Focus on Acute and Chronic Pain

Series edited by
Antonino Gullo

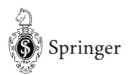 Springer

M.A. TIENGO, MD
Professor Emeritus of Physiopathology and Pain Therapy
State University of Milan, Italy

Series *Topics in Anaesthesia and Critical Care* edited by
A. GULLO, MD
Department of Clinical Science – Section of Anaesthesia,
Intensive Care and Pain Clinic
University of Trieste, Cattinara Hospital, Trieste, Italy

Springer-Verlag Italia
a member of BertelsmannSpringer Science+Business Media GmbH

© Springer-Verlag Italia, Milano 2001

ISBN-13: 978-88-470-0134-3   e-ISBN-13: 978-88-470-2258-4
DOI: 10.1007/978-88-470-2258-4

Library of Congress Cataloging-in-Publication Data: Applied for

This work is subject to copyright. All rights are reserved, whether the whole or part of the material is concerned, specifically the rights of translation, reprinting, re-use of illustrations, recitation, broadcasting, reproduction on microfilms or in other ways, and storage in data banks. Duplication of this publication or parts thereof is only permitted under the provisions of the Italian Copyright Law in its current version, and permission for use must always be obtained from Springer-Verlag. Violations are liable for prosecution under the Italian Copyright Law.

The use of registered names, trademarks, etc. in this publication does not imply, even in the absence of a specific statement, that such names are exempt from the relevant protective laws and regulations and therefore free for general use.

Product liability: the publisher cannot guarantee the accuracy of any information about dosage and application contained in this book. In every individual case the user must check such information by consulting the relevant literature.

Cover design: Simona Colombo
Typesetting and layout: Photo Life, Milan

SPIN: 10790136

Preface

Probably no field of medicine has contributed as much to the understanding of neuroscience as has the study of pain. This has been apparent since the publication of the first texts on pain, of which I cite only two of the most important. The first text dates to 1914. *Anoci-association* by G.W. Crile and W.E. Lower was dedicated to the shock caused by surgical intervention; the authors described how the deleterious effects of this form of shock could be reduced by protecting the individual from pain through a series of analgesic medicines.

The second text is a classic surely known to everybody. It appeared many years later, towards the end of the first half of the 1900s. *Pain Mechanisms* was written by W.K. Livingston, a medical officer of the US Marines Reserve. Upon its publication in 1943, the publishing house Macmillan commented: "The tremendous complexity of the problems related to pain and all sensory perceptions adds to the difficulty of interpreting clinical observations, but at the same time adds to its fascinations. Though physiological laboratories have made contributions of fundamental importance [to the future of clinical medicine], ... the study of the Central Nervous System [is] still a long way from the point at which [our knowledge] can be used to explain such clinical states as *causalgia* or *phantom limb pain*." Those who read that stupendous book certainly remember that the clinical section was preceded by one dealing with basic issues in four chapters: (1) the anatomy of pain, (2) the cutaneous receptor and the concept of specificity, (3) the physiology of pain, and (4) the psychology of pain. In a masterly way, this book laid the foundation for the study of pain, and it is still valid today. In its bibliography, the book cited the great neurophysiologists Adrian (professor of physiology at Cambridge) and Sherrington (professor of physiology at Oxford), both Nobel Prize recipients, and many other neuroanatomists, neurophysiologists and psychologists who made fundamental contributions to the study of pain.

When Professor Antonino Gullo, my great friend and sedulous mentor of APICE, proposed that I coordinate the session "Neuroscience: focus on acute and chronic pain", I was more than honored: I was profoundly pleased. This volume contains the presentations made in that session. The reader has only to browse the table of contents to realize that the arguments discussed in this volume deal with salient points which connect neuroscience with the clinical approaches to acute and chronic pain syndromes. One also immediately notices that the individual chapters have been written by scientists who are protagonists in these fields.

Some readers may not agree that issues related to the treatment of terminally ill patients and to the ethics of such care are relevant in a neuroscience text. Let us not forget that the study of the conscience occupies a central position in neuroscience today, and that it involves two "vertices of observation," to borrow an expression from Mauro Mancia. There is the neurobiological vertex that considers the basic conscience, or rather those functions such as wakefulness, attention, perception, and memory. Associated with this consciousness is a psychological and psychodynamic vertex, which encompasses the consciousness of superior order and the consciousness of self in particular, and that also expresses values of ethics.

My personal contribution to the volume is a commemorative presentation of Camillo Golgi who, at the dawn of neuroscience, with his black reaction, was able to visualize neuronal cells and circuits. This discovery then allowed Ramon y Cajal to trace, for the first time, the neuronal routes of pain and touch with admirable accuracy and precision.

I wish to thank all my colleagues who accepted the invitation to participate in the compilation of this volume and who each offered a masterful scientific contribution. I also thank Springer-Verlag for assuming this great editorial responsibility.

Milan, November 2000

M.A. Tiengo
Honorary Member of
International Association
for the Study of Pain
(IASP)

Contents

Chapter 1 - Camillo Golgi: The Dawning of Neuroscience
M.A. Tiengo 1

Chapter 2 - Neurochemistry of Pain Circuits: Physiological versus Pathological Pain
L. Calzà 9

Chapter 3 - First Affluent Neuron
G. Carli 19

Chapter 4 - The Involvement of the Brainstem Reticular Formation in Pain Processing
C. Desbois, L. Monconduit, L. Villanueva 27

Chapter 5 - The Thalamus and Pain
M.L. Sotgiu 37

Chapter 6 - Naloxone, but not Estradiol, Affects the Gonadectomy-Induced Increase in Hippocampal Cholineacetyltransferase Activity in Male Rats
I. Ceccarelli, A. Scaramuzzino, A.M. Aloisi 43

Chapter 7 - Consciousness and Pain
C.R. Chapman, Y. Nakamura 51

Chapter 8 - Visceral Pain Mechanisms
M.A. Giamberardino, J. Vecchiet, G. Affaitati, L. Vecchiet 59

Chapter 9 - PET-Scan and Electrophysiological Assessment of Neuromodulation Procedures for Pain Control
L. García-Larrea, R. Peyron, F. Mauguière, B. Laurent 71

Chapter 10 - Acute Postoperative Pain Service Models
G. Galimberti, P. Di Marco, A. Conti 87

Chapter 11 - Postoperative Functional Pain Management
F. Nicosia 99

Chapter 12 - Timing for Narcotic Drugs in Terminal Illness
S. Mercadante 105

Chapter 13 - Ethical Decisions in Terminal Illness
D. Kettler, M. Mohr 111

Main Symbols 119

Subject Index 121

Contributors

Affaitati G.
Pathophysiology of Pain Laboratory,
Department of Medicine and Science of Aging "G. D'Annunzio",
University of Chieti, Italy

Aloisi A.M.
Institute of Human Physiology, University of Siena, Italy

Calzà L.
Department of Veterinary Morphophysiology and Animal Production,
(DIMORFIPA), University of Bologna, Italy

Carli G.
Institute of Human Physiology, University of Siena, Italy

Ceccarelli I.
Institute of Human Physiology, University of Siena, Italy

Chapman C.R.
Department of Anaesthesiology, University of Washigton, Seattle, USA

Conti A.
Department of Clinical Science - Section of Anaesthesia,
Intensive Care and Pain Clinic, University of Trieste, Cattinara Hospital, Italy

Desbois C.
INSERM, U-161, Paris, France

Di Marco P.
Department of Clinical Science - Section of Anaesthesia,
Intensive Care and Pain Clinic, University of Trieste, Cattinara Hospital, Italy

Galimberti G.
Department of Clinical Science - Section of Anaesthesia,
Intensive Care and Pain Clinic, University of Trieste, Cattinara Hospital, Italy

García-Larrea L.
Functional Neurology Unit, UPRES-EA 1880,
Claude Bernard University, Lyon, and CERMEP, Lyon, France
(affiliated to the Institut Fédératif de Neurosciences of Lyon)

Giamberardino M.A.
Pathophysiology of Pain Laboratory,
Department of Medicine and Science of Aging "G. D'Annunzio",
University of Chieti, Italy

Kettler D.
Department of Anaesthesiology, Critical Care and Emergency Medicine,
University of Göttingen, Germany

Laurent B.
Pain Centre and Neurology Department, St. Etienne University Hospital, France

Mauguière F.
Functional Neurology Unit, UPRES-EA 1880,
Claude Bernard University, Lyon, France
(affiliated to the Institut Fédératif de Neurosciences of Lyon)

Mercadante S.
Anesthesia and Intensive Care Unit, Pain Relief and Palliative Care Unit,
La Maddalena Clinic for Cancer, Palermo, Italy

Mohr M.
Department of Anaesthesiology, Critical Care and Emergency Medicine,
University of Göttingen, Germany

Monconduit L.
INSERM, U-161, Paris, France

Nakamura Y.
Department of Anaesthesiology, University of Washigton, Seattle, USA

Nicosia F.
Department of Anaesthesia, Intensive Care, Acute Pain Medicine and Emergency,
St. Andrea General Teaching Hospital, La Spezia, Italy

Peyron R.
CERMEP Lyon (affiliated to the Institut Fédératif de Neurosciences of Lyon) and
Pain Centre and Neurology Department, St. Etienne University Hospital, France

Scaramuzzino A.
Institute of Human Physiology, University of Siena, Italy

Sotgiu M.L.
Institute of Neuroscience and Bioimaging, CNR, Segrate, Italy

Tiengo M.A.
Professor Emeritus of Physiopathology and Pain Therapy,
State University of Milan, Italy

Vecchiet L.
Pathophysiology of Pain Laboratory,
Department of Medicine and Science of Aging "G. D'Annunzio",
University of Chieti, Italy

Vecchiet J.
Pathophysiology of Pain Laboratory,
Department of Medicine and Science of Aging "G. D'Annunzio",
University of Chieti, Italy

Villanueva L.
INSERM, U-161, Paris, France

Chapter 1

Camillo Golgi: The Dawning of Neuroscience

M.A. TIENGO

"Even so nervous tissue did not became the subject of a special science until the late 1800s, when the first detailed descriptions of nerve cells were undertaken by Camillo Golgi and Santiago Ramon y Cajal."

Eric R. Kandel [3]

"But in my opinion he was never so grand, for his sharp intuition and his heroic persistence, as when, just 30 years old in a small city of the Milan hinterland, without any help and with rather rudimentary means, he came to discover the "black reaction," by which he was the first to succeed in removing the heavy veil that covered our understanding on the structure of the central nervous system, and it was thereafter possible, as a result of his merit and that of numerous other experimenters, to make further key discoveries in all areas of histology."

Luigi Berzolari,
University of Pavia,
In: Commemoration of Camillo Golgi, November 1926

To establish the date of the birth of neuroscience is difficult and uncertain. In fact, the term "neuroscience" covers a vast range of biological sciences which today

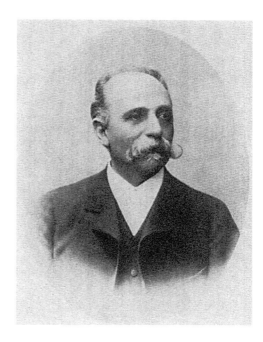

Fig. 1. Camillo Golgi, in 1906, the year of the Nobel Prize

includes various disciplines: anatomy, physiology, neurochemistry, and genetics, as well as psychology and psychiatry. In a word, it includes everything which refers to the nervous system of living beings. Further, it is historically absurd to want to give the role of founder of neuroscience to just one person. Nevertheless, we may affirm that the work of Camillo Golgi amply contributed to the birth of neuroscience, and for this great merit he, together with Cajal, received the Nobel Prize.

Camillo Golgi (Fig. 1) was born on 7 July 1843, at Pisogneto di Corteno, a group of simple little cottages situated near the beginning of the road to Aprica. His father, Alessandro, was a doctor, and his mother, Carolina (the widow of General Papini), was a housewife. He went to elementary and secondary school in Pavia. In 1859, he took part in something which, to say the least, makes one laugh: the 16-years old Camillo was arrested, together with 15 other school companions, for having written something on the city walls which seemed insulting to the occupying Austrians: "Those who study German are spies." In 1860, he enrolled in the faculty of medicine and surgery at the University of Pavia. During the summer session of 1865, Camillo Golgi, only 22-years old, graduated in medicine, having defended a thesis on the aetiology of mental actions; his thesis professor was Cesare Lombroso. In 1876, Camillo Golgi was nominated Professor of Histology at the University of Pavia. Thus, in that year he left the post of Chief Physician which he had occupied since 1872 at the Hospital of Abbiategrasso, in order to move to Pavia where he would live for the rest of his work-filled existence. In 1877, Golgi married Angelina Aletti, the niece of his great friend and mentor, the pathologist Giulio Bizzozzero. The first years of the twentieth-century were triumphal ones for Golgi. In June of 1900, King Umberto the First nominated him Senator for Life for his high scientific merits. Numerous were the recognitions, awards, and nominations which he would have in those years. In 1906, from the Academy of Sweden came the announcement of the bestowal of the Nobel Prize shared equally with him by Ramon Y Cajal (Fig. 2). However, this event did not give Golgi a great deal of pleasure because the two men (more on Golgi's part than on Cajal's) were not on good terms: Golgi accused Cajal of having plagiarized his work on black reaction. The great event of the consignment of the award, therefore, was darkened by these feelings of incomprehension. Another event embittered not only just a little the last years of Golgi's life: the founding of the University of Milan which, for Golgi, greatly diminished the centuries-old prestige of the University of Pavia.

Golgi's Discoveries

The name of Camillo Golgi is tied to many anatomical and physiological discoveries, but at least four are of great importance: black reaction (argentic impregnation of neurons), musculotendinous nerve-ending organs, individuation of type I and type II neurons, and the diffuse neuronal net. I will limit myself to refer only to the first two because the first represented the principal merit of the Nobel Prize awarded to Golgi and Cajal (the Spanish anatomist who adopted and perfected the argentic colouring procedure in order to complete a gigantic study on the histol-

Fig. 2. Ramon Y Cajal

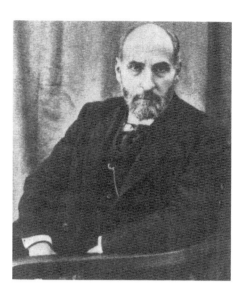

ogy of the nervous system of men and vertebrates), and I believe the second is of utmost importance.

Giacomo Goldaniga [1] writes, "In the winter of 1873, at Abbiategrasso, Golgi made his principal discovery: black reaction, named also chromo-argentico, or the method of Golgi. Already a few years earlier, when he was working at Pavia, he was seeking new methods of colouring nerve tissue in order to succeed in throwing into relief the cellular structure. Before his revolutionary discovery, the preparations to examine under the microscope were coloured either with artificial chemical substances, like picric acid, magenta, aniline blue, or Paris blue, or with natural colorants, like saffron, mallow of Perkin, hematoxylin, and carmine. This last was the most commonly adopted because, among all the substances, it gave the most appreciable results. Golgi, after various attempts, and after having hardened the nervous tissue with potassium bichromate, substituted the carmine with nitrate of silver with the result that the nerve cells were impregnated with silver chromate, revealing themselves for the first time with all their edges precise and well-defined, and with all their ramifications. One could even see the fibres at a considerable distance from their point of origin, so that the new coloration permitted a topographical description of the various groups of nerve cells, and made possible the beginning of modern neuroanatomy and neurohistology."

Golgi's second great discovery – published from 1878 to 1880 – which we will consider refers to the sensitive corpuscles at the ends of the tendons. Goldaniga [2] writes, "This study was of great interest because in that epoch there was a gap between what the clinical, psychophysical, and physiological experiments lead to believe, and that which the few anatomical studies had demonstrated. In essence, one knew that the nerves penetrated into the tendons, but one had no precise idea about how they ended... To clarify this problem could furnish indications on the interpretation of the sensitive base of motility. For a long time, one knew that hitting a tendon produced a rapid contraction of the corresponding muscle, but one didn't know why this occurred. Golgi confronted the problem from a comparative anatomy point of view, and studied the tendons of humans and other vertebrates. Not content with a superficial study, Golgi examined the entire tendon from its attachment to the bone to its muscular insertion, and pushed himself to arrive where no one else ever had, arriving at the deepest layers of the tendon, where the nerve fiber is distributed in its end-most nerve branches among the fascicles of the tendons near to its junction with the muscle." In this area, the first two arboreous corpuscles appeared to him in such form, aspect, and structure that, in Golgi's own words, they were not comparable to any nerve body known today. To these, because of the relationship which they have with muscles on the one hand, and with tendons on the other, the name musculotendinous nerve ending organs must be applied" (Fig. 3).

The development of neuroscience has clarified the important function of these neural formations. In the third edition of Kandel which was published only a few weeks ago, one reads, "Golgi tendon organs are sensory receptors located at the junction between muscle fibres and tendon; they are therefore connected in series to a group of skeletal muscle fibres. These receptors are slender, encapsulated structures about 1 mm long and 0,1 mm in diameter. Stretching of the tendon organ straightens the collagen fibres, thus compressing the nerve endings, and causing them to fire. Whereas muscle spindles are most sensitive to changes in length of a

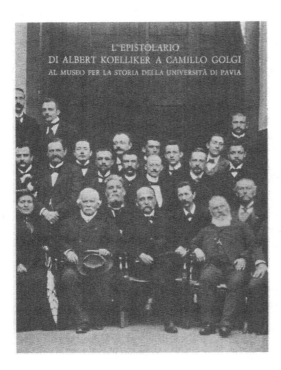

Fig. 3. Congress of Anatomy on Neuron Theory, at the University of Pavia, the 21st of April, 1900. Camillo Golgi is in the *center*. Next to him on his *left* is Koelliker, on his *right* Waldejer

muscle, tendon organs are most sensitive to changes in muscle tension. A particularly potent stimulus for activating a tendon organ is a contraction of the muscle fibres connected to the collagen fiber bundle containing the receptor. The tendon organs are thus readily activated during normal movements. Golgi tendon organs were originally thought to have a protective function, preventing damage to muscle, since it was assumed that they fired only when high tensions were achieved. But we now know that they also signal minute changes in muscle tension, thus providing the nervous system with precise information about the state of contraction of the muscle. The convergence of afferent input from tendon organs, cutaneous receptors, and joint receptors onto interneurons that inhibit motor neurons may allow for precise spinal control of muscle tension in activities such as grasping a delicate object. Combined input from these receptors excites the Ib inhibitory interneurons when the limb contacts the object and so reduces the level of muscle contraction to permit an appropriate soft grasp"[3]. The second type of nerve corpuscle endings, better known as Golgi-Bazzoni bodies, are found on the surface of tendons, and were considered by Golgi as tactile bodies, sensitive, having in common with the corpuscles of Pacini the translation of pressure stimulation.

The Theory of the Neuron in the Thought of Golgi

On the evening of 11 December 1906, Camillo Golgi received from the hands of the Swedish sovereign the maximum recognition for scientific merits: the Nobel Prize. In his Nobel lecture, entitled "The Doctrine of the Neuron. Theory and Fact" [4], he surprised everyone by completely contradicting the theory of the neuron proposed by Cajal, who became furious. Golgi's lecture was divided into three parts. The first part discusses the fact that the neuron may be an embryological unit, that is to say, that it may derive from a single embryonic cell. "That which I have espoused up to now," writes Golgi, "I believe may justify the affirmation that, given the actual state of knowledge about the histogenesis of the nervous system, it is not possible to affirm with confidence that which is known about the origin of the nerve cells may be taken as a fundamental keystone, certain, as the affirmed embriologycal independence of the nerve cell." The second part supports the thesis that "the neuron is, also in the adult state, an independent cellular unity." It demonstrates that the entire elementary nerve apparatus may be considered as an independent anatomical unit. The third part, in my opinion, is the most interesting in that it represents the neuro-biological thought of Golgi, and, therefore, I cite it more extensively. Golgi sets himself the task of demonstrating that the neuron is an independent physiological unit. Golgi writes, "The doctrine of the functional independence of the neuron would have been able to find indirect support in the studies of the so-called cerebral localizations, if granted that the concept of the localizations were maintained in the initial form, that of the precise functions of sense and of motion being assigned to well determined and defined regions of the brain. However, by now the ideas on localization are being modified profoundly. Setting aside the experimental data, such as the possible substitutions and compensations, and the undefined confines of the central zones excitable purely anatomically, a prejudicial question arises immediately which I have posed since the very beginning of my studies. Considering these relationships, we may not be of the conviction that, for example, a single nerve fiber may have relationships with an infinite number of nerve cells and with very different parts and being rather far from the nerve centres. It is superfluous to say that, speaking of territories prevalently of distribution it is understood that these gradually merge into other regions in which they prevalently mix themselves with other fascicles of fibres. These observations of an anatomical type may, regarding localizations, more or less completely be translated into a physiological reasoning. Regarding the specific function of the central nervous system, meanwhile, I repeatedly have had to exclude that it may be joined to specific nerve centres; I could not avoid bringing myself to the idea that the specific central function may be related not specifically to the central organization, but to the specificity of the peripheral organs destined to gather, and to transmit the impressions, or to the particular structure of peripheral organs, to which central stimulation is directed. This presentation, of necessity abbreviated, by me regarding the doctrine of the neuron leads to a conclusion which brings me to the point of departure, that is, that none of the arguments on which Waldejer has imposed his affirmation on the individuality and independence of the neuron may resist criticism. As it is said regarding the functional mechanism, far from being able to accept the idea of the individuality and independence of the single nerve elements, until now I have found no motive for distancing myself from the idea which I have expressed insistently that the nerve cells, rather than an individual action, instead act together, leading to the need to think that many groups of elements may exert a cumulative action on peripheral organs with entire fascicles of fibers in between, one understands that this concept leads also to an inverse action regarding sense actions. As much as I may bang against the diffused tendency individualizing the nerve elements, I do not know how to move from the thought of a unitary action of the nervous system, nor does this worry me if this brings me to an ancient concept! The find which I discovered on the foot of the hippocampus documents in the most objective manner, I would say almost schematically, and it has nothing to do with schema this my method of understanding cellular action of the different provinces of the central nervous system."

These are the concepts and the criteria which for an entire life guided the work of Camillo Golgi, and, re-read today after a century, continue to move and surprise us. In this reading is seen clearly the direction which Golgi's research gave to the development of the knowledge of the nervous system (Fig. 4).

Epilogue

Camillo Golgi, teaching us for the first time aspects which until then were unknown about the anatomy and physiology of the neuron, laid one of the first stones in the immense and stupendous edifice which today we call neuroscience. We were at the beginning of a century which saw neuroscience make unimaginable progress. The scientific richness accumulated in the preceding century was there, all to develop. Camillo Golgi, a truly great genius, sure of himself and of the roads

Fig. 4. Sensorial pathways of touch and pain in a drawing by Ramon Y Cajal

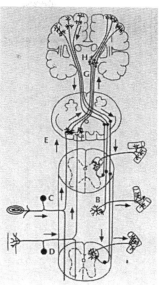

which he traversed, knew how to do it. One day in 1923, Golgi (who would die in 1926) said to a friend, "One has just arrived at the beginning of the knowledge of the mysteries of life, and already one must leave it."

References

1. Goldaniga G (1997) Storia Illustrata di Camillo Golgi, Carpeno Golgi, Brescia, p 29
2. Goldaniga G, Marchetti G (1994) Vita ed opere dello scienziato e Senatore Camillo Golgi (Premio Nobel per la medicina nel 1906). Istituto Bresciano per la Ricerca Biomedica, Brescia, pp 94-95
3. Kandel ER, James H Schwartz JH, Thomas M. Jessel TM (2000) Principles of neural science, 4th edn. McGraw Hill, New York, p 723 and Box 36-3, p 724
4. Golgi C (1907) La doctrine du Neurone, Theorie e Faits, Imprimirie Royal, P.-A. Norstedt & Fils

Suggested Readings

Barker RA (1991) Neuroscience, an illustrated guide; Ellis Horwood, New York
Brazier AB (1984) A History of Neurophysiology in the 17th and 18th centuries. Raven, New York, pp 3
Delcomyn F (1996) Foundations of neurobiology. Freeman, New York
Gregory RL (1987) The Oxford companion of the mind. Oxford University Press, Oxford
Tiengo MA (ed) (1999) Il dolore: una sfida nelle neuroscienze e nella clinica, Springer, Milano, Berlin
Tiengo MA (ed) (2000) Il dolore e la mente. Springer Milano, Berlin

Chapter 2

Neurochemistry of Pain Circuits: Physiological versus Pathological Pain

L. CALZÀ

In the last 15 years, human and animal studies have indicated that the anatomical, neurochemical and functional correlates of pain states are quite different in symptomatic and pathologic pain [1, 2]. Thus, the biological substrate for pharmacological therapy is different for treating acute, symptomatic pain and different types of pathologic chronic pain. Moreover, the pathophysiology of a long-lasting pain syndrome also changes with the course of a disease.

Recent discoveries about neurochemical substrates have enlarged the panel of possible targets for pharmacological therapies. Nitric oxide (NO) as a partner of glutamatergic and peptidergic transmission in pain circuits, nerve growth factor (NGF) in hypersensitivity, ion channels as transducers not only in acute but also in chronic pain (through genomic effects mediated by voltage-dependent channels), and new peptide-mediated analgesia systems are all emerging fields in pain research. At the same time, the genetic aspects of pain perception and suffering have been identified as fundamental not only for individual variability in pain sensitivity and pain pathology development, but also as a possible basis for screening drug sensitivity and for placebo effect (Table 1).

Pain perception may be altered either by the overstimulation of primary afferent fibers or due to a lesion of the neuronal pathway. The first condition is typical in tissue injury and inflammatory pain; the second one is typical for neuropathic pain.

Table 1. Genomic influence in pain threshold and pathology

Human genome research has also produced profond effects on pain research. Genetic influence on pain percepetion, analgesic drugs sensitivity, and occurence of pathologic pain has been recognized, and candidate genes to be inserted in protocols for genetic screening are under study.
- Gender
  - Sex-related incidence of pain syndromes (headache)
- Strains
  - Stress analgesia in different mice strains
  - Deficiency of P450IID6 in 10% of Caucasian population
- Genes
  - Individual pain '"perception"
  - Placebo effect
  - Individual sensitivity to drugs

Incidence of neuropathic pain after deaffentation

10   L. Calzà

Anatomical, functional, and molecular mechanisms in these conditions are quite different, including, for example, long-lasting molecular and behavioral consequences. Some of the most recent development in anatomy, physiology, neurochemistry and molecular biology of primary somatosensory afferences in physiological conditions, in inflammatory and neuropathic pain will be reviewed in this chapter.

Anatomy-Physiology of Primary Sensory Neurons and Spinal Circuit

Primary sensory neurons are pseudo-unipolar neurons with two ending processes, one extending into the peripheral tissues and one projecting to the external layers of the spinal cord, thus representing a bridge between periphery and central nervous system. Nociceptive neurons act not only as conductors of peripheral noxious stimuli to the central nervous system, but their antidromic activation induces the release of active substances in peripheral tissues, e.g., vasoactive compounds, which are responsible for so-called neurogenic inflammation (Fig. 1). The pre-

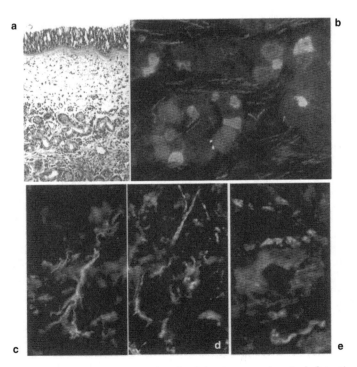

Fig. 1a-e. Primary sensory neurons, visualized by immunochemical detection of substance P in the dorsal root ganglia (**a**) densely innervate peripheral tissues, including superior airways (**b**) hematoxiline-eosin staining of human nasal mucosa); sensory fibers, visualized by immunodetection of the structural protein PGP 9.5 in human larynx, are grouped in small trunks (**c**) or innervate glands (**d**) and blood vessels (**e**) as single fibers

dominant excitatory transmitter in small diameter neurons in DRG is glutamate. Acute pain is generated to a large extent by the release of glutamate that evokes fast synaptic potentials in dorsal horn neurons by activating the AMPA-type glutamate receptor. Substance P (SP), the most investigated substance as transmitter in primary sensory neurons [3], enhances and prolongs the action of glutamate by eliciting slow, excitatory postsynaptic potentials. Substance P and the coexisting peptide calcitonin gene-related peptide (CGRP) are massively released in peripheral tissues when the primary sensory neurons are activated through the classic axon reflex. These peptides cause a degranulation of mast cells and thus the release of histamine, vasodilatation, and plasma extravasation, with the subsequent release of other algogens (bradykinin, serotonin) and the activation of other inflammatory cells (macrophages, monocytes and lymphocytes). Furthermore, substance P induces NO production from the endothelial layer of blood vessels.

Although the previously mentioned concepts have represented the basis of our understanding over the past years, recent studies using transgenic mice have changed some aspects of our view on the role of peptides in pain generation. For example, studies in mice in which the preprotachykinin-A gene has been deleted have indicated that SP contributes to intensity coding only when a stimulus is very intense, thus having a major role in pathological pain [2]. Mice modified for opioid receptor expression have confirmed a significant role for endogenous opioid-peptide interactions with μ opiate receptors in normal nociceptive processing and the role of μ receptor mediation of morphine-induced analgesia in tests of spinal and supraspinal analgesia [4-6].

The peripheral ending of primary sensory neurons acts as a nociceptor. Despite the progress in understanding the molecular mechanisms of signal transduction in other sensory modalities (vision, auditory and olfactory perception), the nature of somatosensory transduction and molecular triggers, with regard to mechanical and thermal stimuli, is still poorly understood (see [7] for a review). Although one hypothesis suggests that mechanical transduction occurs via accessory cells associated with some sensory nerve endings (e.g., Merkel cells and Pacini corpuscles), the "free nerve endings" of nociceptors are not associated with any recognizable accessory structure. Stretch-activated ion channels have been proposed as relevant transducers in high threshold mechanoceptors, but only one mechanosensitive channel in *Escherichia coli* has been cloned so far. Thermal transduction is even more mysterious. However, heat-activated non-selective cation currents have been recorded in cultured dorsal root ganglion neurons.

A subset of chemically defined fibers may be present in C or Aδ fibres. Besson defined the multitude of molecules and related receptors in primary afferent fibers and neurons as a "peripheral jungle" [8]. Help in understanding this jungle, or maybe as a source for making the jungle even more intricate, comes from cloning studies performed using different strategies, which have provided an impressive growth in our knowledge of the receptors and ion channels involved in primary sensory neuron activity [9]. A wide range of receptors for neuroactive substance have been identified in the primary afferent fibers, grouped by Carlton and Coggeshall [10] into receptors associated with nociceptors (for ATP, neurokinin-1, $GABA_A$, $GABA_B$, neuropeptide Y, acetylcholine, somatostatin, prostaglandin E, cholecystokinin, adrenergic, 5HT$_{2A}$ receptor, glutamine, bradykinin, noradrenaline, capsaicin, opioid, angiotensin II, adenosine), those for ligands with non-neuronal sources (acetylcholine, ATP, prostaglandin E, opioids, adenosine, glutamate, bradykinin, noradrenaline, serotonin), and nociceptors (SP, opioid, ATP, adenosine, neuropeptide Y, glutamate, cholecystokinin, somatostatin, bombesin).

After the original identification of an ATP-gated cation channel named P2X3 and the voltage-gated sodium channel SNS in DRG, many more related genes have been cloned, so that 12 different sodium channels in DRG have been identified so far. Moreover, after the original cloning of the VR1 capsaicin receptor, evidence is accumulating in favour of the existence of multiple capsaicin receptors [11]. Related receptors are differentially expressed in peripheral nerve endings vs. axon of unmyelinated C-fibers and myelinated Aδ fibers, thus being differentially associated to the chemical, thermal, and mechanical activation of peripheral nociceptors. Parallel to these genetic and molecular results is the development of channel blockers selective for nociceptive fibers that do not pass the blood-brain barrier and that would also not have any cardiac and central-nervous system depressant effects.

Studies on opioid receptors have also provided new information on the synthesis in DRG neurons, axonal transport in the peripheral and central branches, assembly in the plasma membrane, and the dynamics of internalization.

The neurochemical substrate of pain transmission and control in the spinal cord is also extremely complicated. Possible pharmacological manipulation of pain information entry in the central nervous system is based either on the inhibition of pain transmission (e.g., by blocking substance P and/or glutamate receptors) or an enhancement of endogenous analgesia systems (e.g., through the activation of opioid receptors inhibiting SP release or through the enhancement of the spinal GABAergic system). In fact, pain perception derives from a complex balance between pain transmission and pain inhibition (analgesia) neuronal systems, coupled to supraspinal levels also including limbic and cognitive components (Fig. 2).

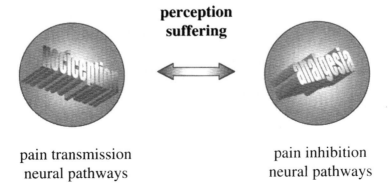

Fig. 2. Pain perception derives from a complex balance between neural systems devoted to pain transmission and pain inhibition (analgesia), coupled to supraspinal levels, also including limbic and cognitive components

In recent years particular attention has been devoted to the role of glutamatergic transmission in pain processing in the spinal cord, also in view of the emerging role of NO in pain. NMDA receptors are important in the synaptic events which lead to central sensitization and hyperalgesia [12, 13]. These phenomena were observed under conditions of severe and persistent injury (see next paragraph), derived by opening of the postsynaptic ion channel-gated NMDA-type of glutamate receptors. The noxious activation can, therefore, produce long-term changes in dorsal horn neurons, similarly to long-term potentiation in the hippocampus, providing a molecular memory trace of C fibers inputs [14]. NO is a modulator of glutamatergic transmission also participating in the development and maintenance of hyperalgesia induced by peripheral inflammation [15]. NO acts as a peripheral mediator of chemically induced nociception, i.e., bradykinin-induced nociception, but results of recent behavioral [15, 16] and electrophysiological [17] experiments have also suggested that the neuronal synthesis of NO in dorsal root ganglia, the spinal cord and supraspinal regions, supports nociceptive transmission and hyperalgesia [18]. NO also modulates the release of sensory neuropeptides in the substantia gelatinosa [19]. Moreover, modulation of NO production by neural cells decreases peripheral inflammation due to adjuvant injection [20].

Pathophysiology of Primary Sensory Neurons and the Spinal Circuit

A number of experimental models of acute and chronic pain in rodents have been developed over the past two decades, and great attention has been devoted to produce "pure" pathogenic events. Thus, using several irritant substances injected in to the peripheral tissues can mimic inflammatory pain, whereas neuropathic pain can be produced by nerve or root constriction models or by transection of peripheral nerves or roots. Both inflammatory and neuropathic states produce increased behavioral responses to noxious stimuli, termed hyperalgesia, and increased nociceptor excitability, termed sensitization (Fig. 3). These phenomena can be generated by the interaction of primary afferent with direct-acting agents (PGE$_2$, PGI$_2$, 8R, 15S-diHETE, serotonin and adenosine), the receptors of which are coupled to G-proteins [7]. This interaction leads to activation of intracellular pathways, including phospholipase C, cAMP, protein-kinase C, but also to alteration in ion current flow. In particular, the available evidence most strongly implicates a Ca^{2+}-dependent potassium current and TTX-R I$_{Na}$ in inflammatory mediator-induced nociceptor sensitization.

Although evidence is accumulating on the modulation of sensory transduction after nerve injury and neuropathy, other mechanisms are believed to play a crucial role in the development of neuropathic pain in chronic nerve injury. In fact, marked changes in neuronal phenotypes in dorsal root ganglia (DRGs) also occur, and these changes may provide clues to the possible mechanisms underlying persistent pain in these experimental models [21-23]. In both inflammatory and neuropathic pain, characteristic regulation of gene expression patterns has

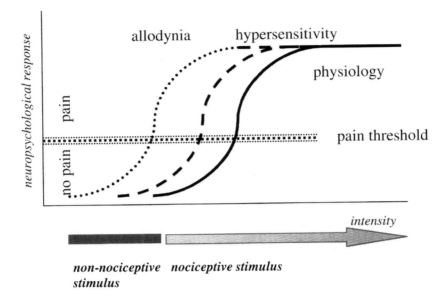

Fig. 3. Alterations in pain perception include hyperalgesia and allodynia. According to pain definitions elaborated by the International Pain Association for the Study of Pain (see http://www.halcyon.com/iasp/defsopen.html), hyperalgesia is "An increased response to a stimulus which is normally painful", whereas allodynia is "Pain due to a stimulus which does not normally provoke pain". These concepts are represented in the graph, which reports the neuropsychological response to stimuli of different intensity and different quality (elaborated from a slide presented by Cervero at the 9th World Congress on Pain, Vienna, Austria, August 22-27, 1999) [see also 24, 25]

been described, both as a consequence of strongly stimulated primary sensory neurons during inflammation [26, 27], as well as of a reduced or lost availability of peripherally derived factors affecting transcription, such as NGF, in neuropathic models [28]. In fact, constant availability of growth factors in normal skin is needed to maintain neuronal phenotype. For example, NGF, which is retrogradely transported from innervation targets to sensory neuron cell bodies, regulates the concentration of neuropeptide transmitters. Traumatic, or chemical, or viral injury of axons initiates profound phenotype changes through disruption of communication between the nerve endings and the cell body.

Changes in peptide synthesis in DRG and the spinal cord after injury of a peripheral nerve or after inflammation are preceded by changes in transcription factors activity, including the early activated genes (IEGs) *c-fos*, *c-jun*, and NF-KB. Transcription factors may contribute to long-lasting changes in pain circuit anatomy and physiology by regulating the synthesis of proteins associated to axonal regrowth, such as GAP-43, or may be responsible for the regulation of the peptide levels seen in neurons after peripheral injury and noxious stimulation (SP, CGRP, neuropeptide Y, etc.) [29]. In the spinal cord, IEGs related proteins also heterodimerize with members of the CREB/ATF family, regulating excitatory (NMDA) receptor synthesis in neuropathic pain models and opioid peptide synthesis during inflammatory pain. Interestingly, long-lasting activation of *c-fos* has been described, raising the question of the meaning of prolonged synthesis of the so-called immediate-early activated genes.

Local environment is also crucial for nerve cell function. In axonal injury, Schwann cells switch from myelin to growth factor production, with profound effects on neurons [30]. After nerve injury, sensory neurons exhibit foci of hyperexcitability and ectopic action potential (due to altered expression of TTX sensitive and insensitive sodium channels). This stimulus-independent pain may be also sympathetically maintained, since after partial nerve injury, injured and uninjured axons begin to express α-adrenoreceptors, which renders them sensitive to circulating catecholamines and norepinephrine released from postganglionic sympathetic terminals [31]. Moreover, a decreased functional tone of inhibitory systems in the spinal cord may also involved in neuropathic pain [32]. GABA and cholecystokinin are believed to play a major role in central "disinhibition".

Mechanical hyperalgesia is one of the most common manifestations of neuropathy. Because of central sensitization due to the continuous input to the dorsal horn, innocuous stimuli that would normally be innocuous are now painful. Clifford Woolf has indicated that a complete anatomical and molecular re-organization in the synaptic circuitry of the dorsal horn after peripheral nerve injury sustains tactile allodynia [28, 33] ("marker hypersensitivity to stimuli that would usually evoke an innocuous sensation", see also Fig. 3 and Cervero [24, 25]). In this condition, Aβ fibers, which normally generate innocuous sensations, began to produce pain. According to the Woolf, the core of this phenomenon is the sprouting of Aβ fibers, which normally terminate in lamina III, into lamina II after peripheral nerve injury. After peripheral nerve injury, Aβ fibers generate synaptic contacts in the place of the C fibers that normally occupy this area. Allong with this functional change, corresponding, large Aβ neurons in DRG start to produce P. However, Hökfelt et al. [22, 34] indicted that axonal spouting after peripheral axotomy occurs not only for Aβ, but also for C fibers; thus, the concept of sprouting in the dorsal horn after peripheral nerve injury needs to be re-evaluated.

Finally, mixed inflammatory and neuropathic conditions also exist and these are prevalent in clinical practice [35, 36]. In cancer pain, for example, inflammatory pain can predominate during early stages of the disease, but when local tumor invasion has taken place, peripheral nerves or terminal branches may be injured, causing neuropathic pain. Similarly, in non-malignant conditions, such as rheumatoid arthritis, synovial innervation is reduced and even eliminated, when the disease progresses and synovial growth spreads to joint soft tissue and attacks bone [37]. This also implies that the general assumption on reversibility of inflammation-related alteration of nociceptor sensitivity and excitability should be considered with caution.

Galanin as Novel Analgesic Peptide in Dorsal Root Ganglia

The role of peptides in pain transmission and modulation is under extensive investigation also from the perspective of new drug development. Recently, much attention has been devoted to galanin, a 29-amino acid peptide originally discovered by Tatemoto and Mutt in the porcine gut [38]. Galanin is widely distributed in the rat brain and spinal cord, where it is synthesized in neurons and, under certain conditions, also by glial cells. In pain circuits, it is expressed in a small population of primary sensory neurons and in interneurons in the superficial dorsal horn in the spinal cord. Galanin receptors have been cloned, and their presence in neurons and glial cells has been described in the rat brain. Galanin is a regulatory peptide implicated in the control of the anterior pituitary function, in feeding and diet preferences. Its role in the physiological process of nociceptive information and in inflammatory and neuropathic pain is under extensive investigation [39]. Galanin synthesis is strongly regulated in DRG neurons after different types of injury of the sciatic nerve, that is, complete nerve transection, nerve constriction and chemical lesion (see [36] for complete references). It has been suggested that galanin plays a tonic inhibitory role in the mediation of spinal cord excitability, and this function is remarkably enhanced after peripheral nerve dissection [21]. Hökfelt et al. [22] have proposed that, whereas opioid local dorsal horn neurons represent a defence system against inflammatory pain, a second defense system, against neuropathic pain, is intrinsic to DRG neurons and utilize galanin as a transmitter peptide. Galanin also interacts with opioids. Intrathecal galanin potentiates the spinal analgesic effect of morphine, and a putative galanin receptor antagonist attenuates opiate and non-opiate analgesia.

References

1. Loeser JD, Melzack R (1999) Pain: an overview. Lancet 353:1607-1609
2. Basbaum AI (1999) Distinct neurochemical features of acute and persistent pain? Proc Natl Acad Sci USA 96:7739-7743
3. Dalsgaard C-J (1988) The sensory system. In: Bjorklund A, Hokfelt T, Owman C (eds) The peripheral nervous system. Handbook of chemical neuroanatomy, vol. 6. Elsevier, Amsterdam, pp 599-636
4. Kieffer BL (1999) Opioids: first lessons from knockout mice. Trends Pharmacol Sci. 20:19-26
5. Matthes HW, Maldonado R, Simonin F et al (1996) Loss of morphine-induced analgesia, reward effect and withdrawal symptoms in mice lacking the mu-opioid-receptor gene. Nature 383:819-23
6. Sora I, Takahashi N, Funada M et al (1997) Opiate receptor knockout mice define mu receptor roles in endogenous nociceptive responses and morphine-induced analgesia. Proc Natl Acad Sci USA 94:1544-1549
7. Tanner KD, Gold MS, Reichling DB, Levine JD (1997) Transduction and excitability in nociceptors: dynamic phenomena. In: Borsook D (ed) Molecular neurobiology of pain. Progress in pain research and management, vol. 9. IASP Press, Seattle, pp 79-105
8. Besson JM (1999) The neurobiology of pain. Lancet 353:1610-1615
9. Wood JN, Akopian AN, Cesare P et al (2000) The primary nociceptor: special functions,

special receptors. In: Devor M, Rowbotham MC, Wiesenfeld-Hallin Z (eds) Proceedings of the 9th World Congress on Pain. Progress in pain research and management. Vol. 16 IASP Press, Seattle, pp 47-62
10. Carlton SM, Coggeshall RE (1998) Nociceptive integration: does it have a peripheral component? Pain Forum 7:71-78
11. Szallasi A, Blumberg PM (1999) Vanilloid (Capsaicin) receptors and mechanisms. (rewiew) Pharmacol Rev 51:159-212
12. Dickenson AH (1995) Spinal cord pharmacology of pain. Br J Anaesth 75:193-200
13. Dickenson AH, Chapman V (2000) New and old anticonvulsants as analgesics. In: Devor M, Rowbotham MC, Wiesenfeld-Hallin Z (eds) Proceedings of the 9th World Congress on Pain. Progress in pain research and management, vol. 16. IASP Press, Seattle, pp 875-886
14. Calzà L, Pozza M, Zanni M (1999) Neurochemical memory in pain circuits. In: Tiengo M, Paladini VA, Rawal N (eds) Regional anaesthesia analgesia and pain management. Basic guidlines and clinical orientation, Springer Milano, pp 23-31
15. Meller ST, Gebhart GF (1993) Nitric oxide (NO) and nociceptive processing in the spinal cord. Pain 52:127-136
16. Malmberg AB, Yaksh TL (1993) Spinal nitric oxide synthesis inhibition blocks NMDA-induced thermal hyperlagesia and produce antinociception in the formalin test in rats. Pain 54:291-300
17. Stanfa LC, Misra C, Dickenson AH (1996) Amplification of spinal nociceptive transmission depends on the generation of nitric oxide in normal and carrageenan rats. Brain Res 737:92-98
18. Urban MO, Gebhart GF (1999) Supraspinal contributions to hyperalgesia. Proc Natl Acad Sci USA 96:7687-7692
19. Aimar P, Pasti L, Carmignoto G, Merighi A (1998) Nitric-oxide-producing islet cells modulate the release of sensory neuropeptides in the rat substantia gelatinosa. J Neurosci 18:10375-10388
20. Pozza M, Bettelli C, Magnani F et al (1998) Is neuronal nitric oxide involved in adjuvant-induced joint inflammation? Eur J Pharmacol 359:87-93
21. Hökfelt T, Zhang X, Wiesenfeld-Hallin Z (1994) Messenger plasticity in primary sensory neurons following axotomy and its functional implications. Trends Neurosci 17:22-30
22. Hökfelt T, Zhang X, Xu X-Q et al (1997) Transition of pain from acute to chronic: cellular and synaptic mechanisms. In: Jensen TS, Turner JA, Wiesenfeld-Hallin Z (eds) Proceedings 8th World Congress on Pain. IASP Press, Seattle, pp 133-154
23. Millan MJ (1999) The induction of pain: an integrated review. Prog Neurobiol 57:1-164
24. Cervero F, Laird JM (1996) Mechanisms of touch-evoked pain (allodynia): a new model. Pain 68:13-23
25. Cervero F, Laird JM (1996) From acute to chronic pain: mechanisms and hypotheses. Prog Brain Res 110:3-15
26 Dubner R, Ruda MA (1992) Activity-dependent neuronal plasticity following tissue injury and inflammation. Trends Neurosci 15:96-103
27. Uhl GR, Nishimori T (1990) Neuropeptide gene expression regulation and neural activity: assessing a working hypothesis in nucleus caudalis and dorsal horn neurons expressing preproenkephalin and preprodynorphin. Cell Mol Neurobiol 10:73-98
28. Woolf CJ (1996) Phenotypic modification of primary sensory neurons: the role of nerve growth factor in the production of persistent pain. Philos Trans R Soc Lond B Biol Sci 351:441-448
29. Doyle CA, Palmer JA, Munglani R, Hunt SP (1997) Molecular consequences of noxious stimulation. In: Borsook D (ed) Molecular neurobiology of pain. Progress in pain research and management, vol. 9. IASP Press, Seattle, pp 145-169

30. Hall SM (1999) The biology of chronically denervated Schwann cells. Ann N Y Acad Sci 883:215-233
31. Baron R, Levine JD, Fields HL (1999) Causalgia and reflex sympathetic dystrophy: does the sympathetic nervous system contribute to the generation of pain? Muscle Nerve 22:678-695
32. Eide PK (1998) Pathophysiological mechanisms of central neuropathic pain after spinal cord injury. Spinal Cord 36:601-12
33. Woolf CJ, Mannion RJ (1999) Neurophatic pain: aetiology symptoms, mechanisms and management. Lancet 353:1959-1964
34. Tong YG, Wang HF, Ju G et al (1999) Increased uptake and transport of cholera toxin B-subunit in dorsal root ganglion neurons after peripheral axotomy: possible implications for sensory sprouting. J Comp Neurol 404:143-158
35. Calzà L, Pozza M, Arletti R et al (2000) Long-lasting regulation of opiate, galanin and other peptides in dorsal root ganglia and spinal cord during experimental polyarthritis. Exp Neurol 164:333-343
36. Calzà L, Pozza M, Zanni M et al (1998) Peptide plasticity in primary sensory neurons and spinal cord during adjuvant-induced arthritis in the rat: an immunocytochemical and in situ hybridization study. Neuroscience 82:575-589
37. Pozza M, Guerra M, Manzini E, Calzà L (2000) A histochemical study of the rheumatoid synovium: focus on nitric oxide, nerve growth factor high affinity receptor and innervation. J Rheumatol 27:1121-1127
38. Tatemoto K, Rökaeus A, Jörnvall H et al (1983) Galanin - a novel biologically active peptide from porcine intestine: FEBS Lett 164:124-128
39. Wiesenfeld-Hallin Z, Bartfai T, Hökfelt T (1992) Galanin in sensory neurons in the spinal cord. Front Neuroendocrinol 13:319-343

Chapter 3

First Affluent Neuron

G. CARLI

General Aspects of Nociceptors

Sensory neurons responding to stimuli capable of producing tissue damage are termed nociceptors and have free nerve endings of either myelinated small-diameter (Aδ) or unmyerlinated (C) fiber axons. They display either single or multiple receptive fields. Nociceptive afferents supply skin, subcutaneous tissue, periosteum, joints, muscles and viscera. Nociceptors also innervate vessels, meninges, and nervi nervorum. Skin, subcutaneous tissue and fascia are supplied by mechanical nociceptor afferents and heat and cold nociceptors; most of Aδ and C nociceptors in primates are mechano-heat sensitive and respond to chemical stimuli as well and are referred to as polymodal nociceptors.

In intact tissues, nociceptors encode stimulus intensity and localization. Very brief noxious stimulation to the skin with a pinprick or application of noxious heat for an instant elicits a double pain response: a first, fast pain that has a pricking quality and lasts less than 50 ms, followed by a painless interval of 1 s or more, after which time a second, slow pain occurs that has a burning quality and lasts more than 1 s. The first pain is mediated by Aδ fibers and the second pain by C fibers.

In primates, Aδ fibers display nociceptors (type IIA) which occur only in hairy skin, have a short-latency adapting response to heat stimulus and are responsible for signaling the first pain sensation to heat [1]: this is in agreement with the absence of a first pain sensation to heat stimuli applied to the glabrous skin of the human hand [2]. A fiber nociceptors in hairy skin and C fiber nociceptors in both skin types are characterized by a fast discharge stimulus onset response, fatigue and adaptation. In rats, fast heating rates to suprathreshold temperatures preferentially activates Aδ nociceptors, whereas slower heating rates activate C-fiber nociceptors.

All Aδ and C fibers in rat hairy skin are excited by noxious cold and their responses increase as stimulus temperature decreases. Many nociceptors are excited only if the stimulus temperatures approach 0 C° and below. C nociceptors contribute to the sensation of dull pain produced by cold stimuli for temperatures above 0° and Aδ nociceptors contribute to pricking pain evoked by a cold stimuli below 0° [3]. More in general, in humans, glabrous skin is fivefold thicker and has more epidermal layers than hairy skin. Cold-induced pain thresholds are lower for the hairy skin of the dorsolateral hand than the glabrous skin of the thenar eminence [4]. Since cold pain in humans can be evoked by cold stimuli applied within the veins and is abolished by a local anesthetic applied within the vein but not in the overlying skin, it is likely that cold pain is served mainly by vascular receptors. Slower cooling rates increasing activity in cold-sensitive nociceptors result in higher psychophysical ratings and decreased suprathreshold indices of pain.

In humans, the pain threshold corresponds to the achievement of a given discharge rate in nociceptors (0.5 impulses/s). Aδ fibers can fire at much higher frequencies than C fibers and, therefore, are more suitable for temporal summation at the level of central synapses. Coupling, i.e., the excitation of one fiber from the action potential activity in another, occurs between C fibers in the normal peripheral nerve. Coupling is bidirectional, involves C polymodal nociceptors, occurs near the axon terminals, and is eliminated by small amounts of local anesthetic at the receptive field. Coupling between nociceptors and sympathetic fibers does not occur.

Nociceptors display several properties which allow them to be particularly suitable to complex and integrated functions. For instance, their response depends upon the nociceptive stimuli previously received and by the condition of the innervated tissues. In fact, axon terminals not only function is energy transductions and generating action potentials but may act as effectors by releasing vasoactive peptides such as substance P and calcitonin gene-related peptide (cGRP), which represent an important nervous system contribution to inflammation.

Sensitization and Inflammation

Following repeated stimulation, nociceptors may become more and more sensitive to an adequate stimulus: such a condition, termed sensitization, is characterized by lowered threshold, decreased response latency, increase in discharge frequency after discharge, and persistence of firing following the end of the external stimulus. At the site of the injury there is primary mechanical and thermal hyperalgesia: the increased sensitivity in uninjured tissue surrounding the lesion is termed secondary hyperalgesia. At the site of the lesion, mechanical hyperalgesia is mainly due to Aδ nociceptors, thermal hyperalgesia to C nociceptors.

Peripheral sensitization does not account for secondary hyperalgesia, where the peripheral signal for pain does not reside exclusively with nociceptors. In these conditions and in neuropathic states, other receptor types, which normally encode the sensation of touch, acquire the capacity to evoke pain. This capacity arises through the augmentation of responsiveness of central pain-signaling neurons to input from low-threshold mechanoceptors, a state often termed "central sensitization".

The main critical protective reaction occurring at the site of a lesion is inflammation. It is characterized by redness and heat which are the result of an increase in blood flow; swelling is the result of increased vascular permeability, and pain is the result of activation and sensitization of nociceptors. Inflammation is a protective process which serves, to insulate the effect of the insult and leads to removal of injured tissue and repair of the injury site.

The most important events leading to activation and sensitization of nociceptors following cell damage are illustrated in Figure 1. Inflammatory mediators include bradykinin (BK), prostaglandins (PGE_2), amines, such as serotonin (5HT)

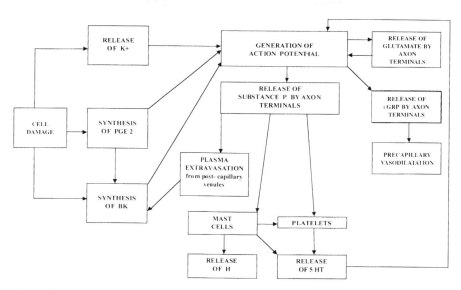

Fig. 1. Schematic view of the interactions between the substances released by the axon terminal and that released by the enjured tissue leading to nociceptor sensitization

and histamine (H), leukotrienes, purines, and cytokines which act on specific targets such as microvasculature, cause the local release of other mediators from leukocytes, and attract other leukocytes to the site of inflammation. Nociceptive neurons also display a peripheral effector role, mediating responses associated with neurogenic inflammation (vasodilation, vascular leakage) via substance P and cGRP and neuroimmune regulation. Many inflammatory mediators directly activate nociceptors and/or contribute to nociceptor sensitization. With sustained peripheral inflammation, prolonged C-fiber activation alters the pattern of gene transcription in dorsal root ganglion (DRG) cells and dorsal horn neurons. Mediators released during inflammation can excite and sensitize nociceptive afferents by acting on ligand-gated ion channels, G-protein-coupled receptors or tyrosine kinase-linked receptors. In addition, some of the sensitizing effects of inflammatory agents may be mediated indirectly by effects on voltage-gated ion channels.

In the inflamed tissue, proton concentration increases and exposure of nociceptors to low pH has been shown to produce sensitization [5]. Proton-sensitive channels, a family of ion channels triggered by increased local acidity, have been recently identified. These proteins, named ASICs (acid-sensing ion channels) consist of five subtypes, each with a distinct pattern of activation kinetics, pH dependence, and tissue specificity. Four of these subtypes are expressed in small-diameter sensory neurons, making them candidate mediators of hyperalgesia in inflamed, poorly perfused tissue that becomes acidotic.

Capsaicin and structurally related molecules bind to specific vanilloid receptors of the peripheral terminals of nociceptive neurons. Receptor occupancy triggers cation influx, action potential firing and the consequent burning sensation associated with spicy food. The cDNA encoding vanilloid-activated cation channel (VR1), that is selectively expressed by small- and medium-diameter neurons within the dorsal root ganglia, has been identified [6]. VR1 can be activated by noxious heat and by protons, both of which excite nociceptors and evoke pain.

It has been recently suggested [7] that heat sensitivity serves a second function, i.e., to sense inflammation and effects of exogenous irritants. This hypothesis postulates that some intracellular mechanisms in the nociceptive terminal lower the heat threshold so that tissue temperature can become a gating force of excitation. The theory suggests a fast sensitizing action of bradykinin which has no direct excitatory effects but lowers the heat threshold in the nociceptor so that the tissue temperature becomes the adequate stimulus to induce the discharge. This could explain the immediate pain relief that results from cooling inflamed, injured, or chemically irritated tissues. Cooling of the skin is also able to abolish pain elicited by infiltration of a buffer solution of low pH or by topical capsaicin application. In conclusion, there is evidence that bradykinin, low pH, as well as several inflammatory mediators act on nociceptors mainly by lowering the threshold of their heat transduction mechanisms, i. e., acting as sensitizers, so that the tissue or the body temperature becomes the driving, adequate stimulus for nociception transduction and pain [7].

Nociceptors normally do not respond to sympathetic stimulation but inflammation may lead to cathecol sensitization of cutaneous nociceptors. It seams that sympathetic efferent activity through $\alpha 2$ receptors may increase the pain associated with inflammation and injury. Opioids, besides their central analgesic effect, become able, within a few hours, to produce analgesia in inflamed tissues by a peripheral mechanism: opioids receptors occur in peripheral terminals of afferent fibers and axonal transport of these receptors is enhanced during inflammation. Inflammatory cells such as macrophages, monocytes, and lymphocytes contain opioid peptides whose release may be induced by interleukin 1β and corticotropin release hormone originating from the inflamed tissue [8]. The local analgesic effect of opioids represents an important plastic mechanism, i.e., occuring for repetitive stimuli, which limits the excitability of nociceptors.

Some tiny myelinated and unmyelinated afferents are not excited by physiological stimuli even at potentially damaging intensities. These neurons, which are insensitive to mechanical stimuli, are called "silent nociceptors" since they develop a responsiveness to mechanical, thermal, and chemical stimuli after exposure to inflammatory mediators. Some of these silent afferents contain neuropeptides which they can liberate under certain circumstances for protective reactions and repair of peripheral tissue. In human hairy skin Schumltz et al. [9] found that some C-fiber afferents had both mechanosensitive and mechanoinsensitive branches: the latter became mechanically excitable after chemical stimulation. Silent afferents are known to supply knee joint, skin and viscera: in the last case they seem to be particularly numerous. It is likely that, when activated, silent nociceptors contribute to pain sensation [9, 10]. Sensitization and recruitment of silent nociceptors represent the main plastic mechanisms which contribute to the amplification of the sensory input.

Sustained subthreshold mechanical stimuli activate various classes of $A\delta$ and C nociceptors, including silent C fibers, and elicit delayed sensations of pain [11]. In particular the latency of pain increases exponentially with decreasing stimulus intensity. This "tarde algesia" differs from hyperalgesia in three respects: it does not involve decrease in nociceptor threshold, it is unaffected by prostaglandin, and it is Ca^{2+} dependent [12].

Neuropathic Pain

Injury and disease affecting peripheral nerves frequently results in the development of chronic "neuropathic" pain. This pain develops with a delay after the injury, can be spontaneous and/or movement-evoked, continuous or paroxysmal, associated with paresthesia, dysesthesia, allodynia, hyperalgesia and hyperpathia. Sometimes it may start as dull pain and become intense or spread from the site of stimulation. In humans, there is no satisfactory medical management for neuropathic pain. Following peripheral nerve injury, changes in neuronal excitability and mRNA levels in sensory neurons offer a substrate for chronic pain. Several mechanisms that contribute to increased excitability in DRG cells have recently been discovered. Nociceptor input triggers and maintains central sensitization whether it arises from inflamed tissue or from ectopic neuropathic sources. In neuropathic pain the development of hyperalgesia can be explained by three different mechanisms which may occur simultaneously (a) central sensitization, (b) peripheral sensitization, and, (c) interaction in the peripheral nerve between injured and intact nerve fibers.

In neuropathic pain ectopic firing may develop: (1) in the nerve region where a trauma or a disease has caused focal demyelination, (2) in DRG cells after axotomy or, (3) in a neuroma that follows a nerve cut. In experimental models, after complete nerve dissection the bulk of the ectopic afferent barrage is generated within the DRG, in the somata rather in the spinal neuroma, and only in A neurons, primarily the non-inflected DRG A_0 type. At the same time some DRG neurons with A-β fibers begin to express substance P and cGRP after injury. Spared DRG neurons also show increased expression of substance P and cGRP that are regulated by NGF. According to their high conduction velocity, the A_0 neurons that become rhythmogenic following axotomy are muscle afferents. It remains to be explained how an input limited to A and excluding C fibers can be the causative factor for triggering central sensitization [13].

After partial nerve injury uninjured primary afferents serving the partially denervated tissue develop abnormal responses and C- fiber nociceptors develop spontaneous activity. Since in animal pain models there is simultaneous emergency, shortly after nerve lesions, of ectopic discharge and tactile allodynia, it is reasonable to assume that ectopic discharges are the causative factor in the development of allodynia. Wallerian degeneration in the periphery alters the environment around intact nerve fibers from adjacent spinal nerve and can represent one of the mechanisms that contribute to neuropathic pain. Wallerian degeneration leads to a local increase in cytokines, NGF, and inflammatory mediators which may affect intact nociceptors and afferent fibers. In conclusion, in partial peripheral nerve lesions, the input from injured nerve fibers plays a critical role in the production and maintenance of central sensitization and hyperalgesia [14].

Axotomy produces a sequence of degenerative events in the sympathetic ganglia and their axons, including shrinkage of cell soma and reduction of axon diameter and conduction velocity. Sympathetic neurons that project to vessels of the DRG start to issue sprouts that invade both dorsal and ventral roots. In the rat DRG, sympathetic sprouts surround the satellite cells that are associated with sensory neurons and form striking basket-like structures. Sprouting of sympathetic fibers can be induced by exogenous application of leukemia inhibitory factor and NGF. The proliferation of sympathetic fibers occurs within days when the spinal nerve is injured close to the DRG and weeks when the nerve is injured more peripherally: it seems that the damaged sensory neurons issue growth signals that attract sympathetic fibers.

The sprouting of sympathetic fibers also involves the contralateral side and is restricted to the homonym segments of the spinal cord. Axotomy elicits bilateral changes in mRNA of cholecystokinin, neuropeptide Y, galanin, vasoactive intestinal polypeptide, and altered expression of opioid and bradykinin binding sites, and these changes are associated with a bilateral increase in NGF [15]. This can account for the numerous reports of bilateral hyperalgesia after unilateral mechanical injury of a peripheral nerve. Nerve injury induces sprouting of sympathetic fibers at the injury site and also in partially denervated skin; nociceptors develop α adrenoceptors and become sensitive to respond directly to noradrenalin so that a direct sympathetic-sensory coupling can exacerbate ectopic firing. After partial nerve injury, both stimulation and norepinephrine injection activate undamaged cutaneous primary afferents [16]. Adrenergic excitation of primary afferents can also occur at the dorsal root ganglion and at the axonal site of injury, and this excitation can be blocked by α antagonists [17]. Appearance of a novel adrenergic responsiveness after partial nerve damage is related to sympathetic denervation of blood vessels and other non-neural tissues: there is evidence that removal of sympathetic innervation to the tissue in which the C-fiber polymodal nociceptors are located induces adrenergic responsiveness [18].

After axotomy, cell death occur in one third of DRG cells but local administration of exogenous NGF may prevent cell death. High-affinity receptors for NGF, trks, which bind to NGF, are expressed by nociceptive afferents and by mast cells. Increased NGF levels occur during inflammation and NGF diplays marked sensitizing actions on nociceptors by producing mast cells degranulation and release of histamine and serotonin and via activation of the 5-lipoxygenase pathway. Blocking NGF bioactivity largely blocks the effects of inflammation on sensory nerve function. NGF administration to adult animals and humans can produce mechanical and thermal hyperalgesia and this effect is abolished by sympathectomy since sympathetic afferents also posses trk receptors. In men and animals, peripheral nerve injury induces adjacent intact cutaneous sensory axons to sprout collateral fibres into the denervated areas for a limited distance. The endogenous NGF can regulate the collateral sprouting of intact nociceptive axons in adult rats after denervation. The collateral sprouting can be blocked by systemic administration of anti-NGF. NGF clearly has powerful neuroprotective effects on small-diameter sensory neurons and its levels change after nerve injury [19].

Sodium (Na) channels open transiently and rapidly when the membrane is depolarized beyond -60 to -40 mV and are responsible for action potential generation and conduction. C cells usually have slow action potentials with a clear inflection on the falling phase. One difference between action potentials in C and A cells is their sensitivity to the blockade by tetrodoxin (TTX): C cells are resistant to the block because they possess a distinct population of TTX-resistant (TTX-R) Sodium channels. SNS is the type of channel responsible for the expression of TTX-R currents. TTX-R activate more slowly, and their currents are activated and inactivated at more depolarized membrane potentials and display a faster rate of recovery from inactivation than TTX-sensitive (TTX-S) channels. In conclusion, TTX-R Sodium currents are particularly able to generate sustained burst of action potentials in response to prolonged depolarizing noxious stimuli [20].

After axotomy, in DRG neurons one channel, type III, which is TTX-S and found only during development, appears to be strongly expressed. In contrast, the TTX-R channel SNS is downregulated after axotomy since SNS expression is controlled by NGF, which is produced by target tissues in the periphery and transported retrogradely to the cell soma. Application of NGF to the damaged nerve endings can reverse this effect. During inflammation there is an increase in production and supply of NGF and an increased expression of TTX-R channels. In general, an increase in Sodium channel density at any region of the neuron may facilitate the action potential generation, particularly in the pattern of prolonged bursts, at that site [21]. It has been suggested that selective blocks of Sodium channels may represent a new therapeutic approach to neuropathic pain.

References

1. Treede RD, Meyer RA, Raja SN, Campbell JN (1995) Evidence for two different transduction mechanisms in nociceptive primary afferents innervating monkey skin. J Physiol 483:747-758
2. Campbell JN, LaMotte RH (1983) Latency to detection of first pain. Brain Res 266:203-208
3. Simone DA, Kajander KC (1997) Responses of cutaneous A-fiber nociceptors to noxious cold. J Neurophysiol 77:2049-2060.
4. Harrison JLK, Davis KD (1999) Cold evoked pain varies with skin type and cooling rate: a psychophysical study in humans. Pain 83:123-135
5. Steen KH, Reeh P, Anton F, Handwerker HO (1992) Protons selectively induce long lasting excitation and sensitization to mechanical stimulation of nociceptors in rat skin, in vitro. J Neurosci 12:86-95
6. Caterina JM, Schumacher MA, Tominaga M, et al (1997) The capsaicin receptor: a heat-activated ion channel in the pain pathway. Nature 389:816-824
7. Reeh PW, Petho G (2000) Nociceptor excitation by thermal sensitization- a hypothesis. In: Sandkuler J, Gebart GF, Bromm B (eds) Nervous System Plasticity and Chronic Pain. Progress in Brain Research Elsevier, Amsterdam (in press)
8. Herz A (1996) Peripheral opioid analgesia-facts and mechanisms. In: Carli G, Zimmermann M (eds) Towards the Neurobiology of Chronic Pain. Progress in Brain Research, vol 110. Elsevier, Amsterdam, pp 95-110

9. Schmeltz M, Schmidt R, Ringkamp M, et al (1994) Sensitization of insensitive branches of C nociceptors in human skin. J Physiol 480:389-394
10. Michaelis M, Habler H-G, Janig W (1997) Silent afferent neurons:a separate class of primary afferents? Clin Exp Pharmacol Physiol 23:99-105
11. Adriaensen H, Gybels J, Handwerker HO, Van Hees J (1984) Nociceptor discharges and sensation due to prolonged noxious mechanical stimulation-a paradox. Hum Neurobiol 3:53-58
12. White DM, Taiwo YO, Coderre TJ, Levine JD (1991) Delayed activation of nociceptors:correlation with delayed pain sensations induced by sustained stimuli. J Neurophysiol 66:229-234
13. Liu C-N, Wall PD, Ben-Dor E, et al (2000) Tactile allodynia in the absence of C-fiber activation:altered firing properties of DRG neurons following spinal nerve injury. Pain 85:503-521
14. Li Y, Dorsi MJ, Meyer RA, and Belzberg AJ (2000) Mechanical hyperalgesia after an L5 spinal nerve lesion in the rat is not dependent on input from injured nerve fibers. Pain 85:493-502
15. Koltzenburg GM, Wall PD, McMahon SB (1999) Does the right side know what the left is doing?. Trends Neurosci 22:122-127
16. Sato J, Perl ER (1991) Adrenergic excitation of cutaneous pain receptors induced by peripheral nerve injury. Science 251:1608-1610
17. Devor M, Seltzer Z (1999) Pathophysiology of damaged nerves in relation to chronic pain. In: Wall PD, Melzack R (eds) Textbook of pain. Churchill Livingston, London, pp 129-164
18. Bossut DF, Shea VK, Perl ER (1996) Sympathectomy induces adrenergic excitability of cutaneous C-Fiber nociceptors. J Neurophysiol 75:514-517
19. McMahon SB, Bennet DLH (1994) Trophic factors and pain. In: Wall PD, Melzack R (eds) Textbook of pain. Churchill-Livingston, Edinburgh, pp 105-128
20. Elliott JR (1997) Slow Na+ channel inactivation and bursting discharge in a simple model axon: implications for neuropathic pain. Brain Res 754:221-226
21. Devor M, Govrin-Lippmann R, Angelides K (1993) Na+ channel immunolocalization in peripheral mammalian axons and changes following nerve injury and neuroma formation. J Neurosci 13:1966-1992

Chapter 4

The Involvement of the Brainstem Reticular Formation in Pain Processing

C. Desbois, L. Monconduit, L. Villanueva

In addition to spinal pathways carrying nociceptive information directly to the diencephalon, some such information is relayed within the caudal brainstem. Indeed, it has been known for a long time that the majority of ascending axons located in the anterolateral quadrant of the spinal white matter, which contains the pain pathways in mammals, terminate within the medullary reticular formation [1-3]. Interestingly, the notion of a receptive centre (*centrum receptorium* or *sensorium*) within the reticular formation was introduced by Kohnstamm and Quensel [4] for bulbar reticular areas receiving spinal afferents. In a study of retrograde cellular reactions in the bulbar reticular formation to high mesencephalic lesions, the same authors demonstrated ascending pathways connecting the *centrum receptorium* with higher levels of the brain. They postulated that reticulo-thalamic projections might be part of a polysynaptic path responsible for the conduction of pain and temperature to higher brain levels [5].

A Caudal Medullary Reticular Region Selectively Activated by Widespread Noxious Inputs

Several groups have shown that widespread areas throughout the brainstem reticular formation contain neurones responsive to noxious stimuli [6-8] and that focal stimulation of some bulbar reticular areas can elicit escape behaviour [9, 10]. However, the way in which the reticular structures participate in the processing of nociceptive information was not clear. This was because reticular units activated by noxious stimulation showed irregular responses and changes in excitability, had receptive fields which were difficult to define and presented some degree of heterosensory convergence. As a result, it was stated that the reticular formation did not play a specific role in the processing of pain.

This proposal has been challenged by data obtained in the rat showing that a well-delimited area within the caudal-most aspect of the medulla, the *subnucleus reticularis dorsalis* (SRD), can play a selective role in processing cutaneous and visceral nociceptive inputs [8]. The SRD region extends caudo-rostrally from the spinomedullary junction to the level of the area postrema and, as shown in Figure 1, lies ventral to the cuneate nucleus and medial to the magnocellular layer of trigeminal nucleus caudalis, and is separated from the subnucleus reticularis ventralis by an acellular boundary extending from the solitary tract to the dorsal border of the lateral reticular nucleus [11-13].

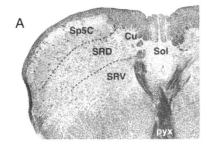 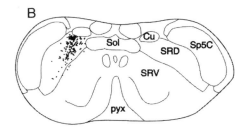

Fig. 1. A Brightfield image of a section of the medulla caudal to the obex stained with the Kluver and Barrera technique. The *dotted line* represents the delimitation of the SRD area with regard to the surrounding trigeminal, SRV and cuneate regions (adapted from [8]). **B** Schematic representation of a coronal section of the medulla, caudal to the area postrema (diagram adapted from [13-55]). Each *dot* represents the recording site of a unit with "whole body" nociceptive convergence. Note that the population is confined within the *subnucleus reticularis dorsalis* (adapted from [8]). *Cu*, cuneate nucleus; *Sol*, nucleus of the solitary tract; *SRD*, *subnucleus reticularis dorsalis*; *SRV*, *subnucleus reticularis ventralis*; *Sp5C*, spinal trigeminal nucleus caudalis; *pyx*, pyramidal decussation

For many years, the SRD was considered to be part of the trigeminal nucleus caudalis. However, the SRD neurones respond exclusively to the activation of Aδ and C fibres from any part of the body surface (Fig. 2A) [14, 15], encode both cutaneous [16] and visceral [17] nociceptive inputs (Fig. 2B, C), and their C-fiber components exhibit the "wind-up" phenomenon during repetitive stimulation. Additional data obtained in the monkey has demonstrated that there are neurones with similar features to those described in the rat SRD. Medullary units recorded in monkeys exhibited convergence of nociceptive inputs from widespread areas of the body and encoded the intensities of peripheral noxious stimuli [18]. Thus, it seems that in different species, dorsal medullary reticular neurones might constitute a morphofunctional entity which processes nociceptive inputs.

The Interactions Between the SRD and the Spinal Cord

The spinal pathways responsible for the activation of SRD neurones ascend via crossed pathways in the lateral aspect of the anterolateral quadrant [19], a region that classically has been implicated in the transmission of messages from a painful focus, as shown by the relief of pain produced by anterolateral cordotomy [20]. However, the fact that the most spinal afferents to the SRD originate from the upper ipsilateral cervical cord, and far fewer from bilateral caudal spinal segments [21, 22], is in contrast to the whole body receptive fields with a contralateral dominance of SRD neurones [14]. This suggests that some of the spinal inputs do not reach the SRD directly. As an alternative, the ascending information may be relayed

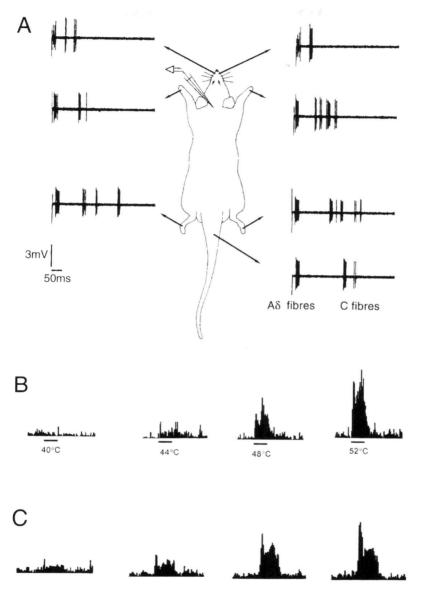

Fig. 2. A Single sweep recordings showing Aδ and C-fiber evoked responses of a SRD neurone following supramaximal percutaneous electrical stimulation of different areas of the body (arrows). Note that massive Aδ and C-fiber responses were evoked from all body areas (adapted from [14]). **B** Discharges of a SRD neurone elicited by graded thermal stimulation of the extremity of the contralateral hindpaw. Note the monotonic increase of the number of spikes per second, within a noxious (44-52°C) range (adapted from [16]). **C** Discharges of a SRD neurone elicited by colo-rectal distensions. The distending pressures are shown beneath each graph. Note the monotonic increase in the neuronal responses within the 25-100 mm Hg range (adapted from [17])

at upper cervical levels which contain both the majority of spino-reticular afferents and neurones with heterosegmental, widespread receptive fields [23, 24]. Interestingly, the largest numbers of retrogradely labelled cells in the spino-thalamic and spino-mesencephalic tracts in the rat were also found to be in the upper cervical cord, thus suggesting a common functional organisation of several ascending somatosensory pathways (see references in [25]). Inputs to the cervical enlargement can originate from different sources, including from collaterals of ascending axons. Within the framework of this hypothesis, one could envisage that at least some inputs to SRD neurones have relays in the upper cervical cord. Together with the fact that other tracts involved in the transmission of nociceptive information may have a similar organisation, this could explain the widespread relief of pain, including pain from caudal segments of the body, following commissural myelotomies of the upper cervical spinal cord in humans [26-30].

Moreover, the spinal neurones that project to the SRD in turn receive descending projections from this area [31-34]. Such reciprocal projections suggest that the SRD participates in spino-reticulo-spinal loops triggered by nociceptive inputs. In this respect, both in animals and in man, the phenomena termed diffuse noxious inhibitory controls (DNIC, see references in [35]) which probably underlie the analgesic effects elicited by acupuncture [36] have shown many functional analogies with the electrophysiological properties of SRD neurones. DNIC are elicited exclusively by noxious inputs; they involve a loop, including the ventrolateral and dorsolateral funiculi as the ascending and descending pathways, respectively; and they act on dorsal horn convergent neurones which are located in areas to which SRD neurones project. Furthermore, SRD lesions strongly reduce DNIC [37], which is reminiscent of the disappearance of DNIC in human subjects with unilateral lesions of the retro-olivary portion of the medulla (Wallenberg's syndrome, [38]).

The Interactions Between the SRD, the Thalamus and the Cortex

The SRD send dense ascending projections to the lateral half of the ventromedial (VMl) thalamus and the lateral aspect of the parafascicular nucleus [39]. VMl thalamic neurones are exclusively driven by activities in Aδ and C-cutaneous polymodal nociceptors from the entire body surface [40]. These neurones present "whole body" receptive fields which are activated by graded stimuli, and a linear relationship exists between the evoked firing rate and the intensities of both thermal and mechanical stimuli only within noxious ranges (Fig. 3B). Finally, in some cases, VMl neurones develop residual activity and/or after-discharges following strong noxious stimulation.

Nociceptive activity in the VMl thalamus arises primarily from monosynaptic inputs from the medullary SRD, since a strong reduction in VMl responses was obtained following blockade of the contralateral SRD (Fig. 3C). As shown above, the SRD is a principal target for afferents from the deep dorsal horn [21, 32], contains most of the neurones with heterosegmental nociceptive convergence [14] and projects densely to the contralateral VMl thalamus [39].

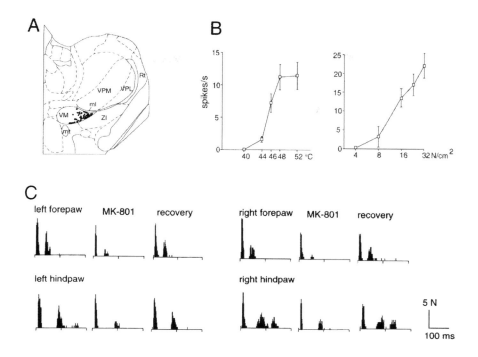

Fig. 3. A Distribution of neurones recorded in the ventromedial thalamic nucleus (VM) that responded to noxious cutaneous stimuli from the entire body surface. Each neurone is presented as a *dot* in a schematic representation of a coronal section of the diencephalon [55]. Note that most of the units recorded were located in the lateral half of VM (VM*l*). Abbreviations: *ml*, medial lemniscus; *mt*, mammillothalamic tract; *Rt*, reticular thalamic nucleus; *Po*, posterior thalamic nucleus; *VM*, ventromedial thalamic nucleus; *VPL*, ventroposterolateral thalamic nucleus; *VPM*, ventral posteromedial thalamic nucleus; *ZI*, zona incerta. **B** Cumulative results showing the magnitudes of the responses of VM*l* neurones to graded mechanical ($n = 7$) or thermal ($n = 16$) stimulation of the ipsilateral hindpaw. **C** Example of the effects of a microinjection of a NMDA antagonist (MK-801) into the left SRD, on the responses of a neurone recorded in the right VM to supramaximal percutaneous electrical stimulation of the four limbs (adapted from [40])

VM*l* neurones in turn relay the widespread nociceptive inputs from the SRD to the whole layer I of the dorsolateral neocortex (Fig. 4). VM projections are organised as a widespread, dense band covering mainly layer I of the dorsolateral anterior-most aspect of the cortex [41]. This band diminishes progressively as one moves caudally, disappearing completely at 1 mm caudal to bregma level. In all mammals, the pyramidal cell – the main output neuron in the neocortex – invariably has its apical dendrites contacting layer I [42, 43]. These findings provide an anatomical and functional basis for any signal of cutaneous pain to alter cortical activity in a universal way, namely by contacting the distal ends of apical dendrites of pyramidal cells in layer I. Thus, the VM*l* thalamus may constitute an important

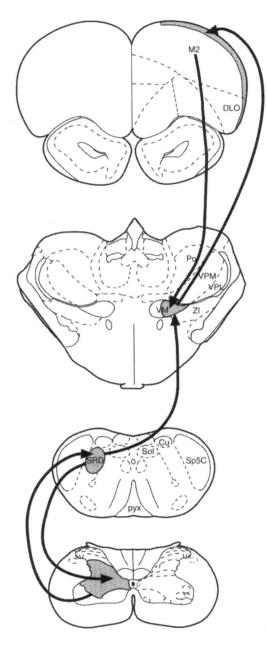

Fig. 4. The integrative role of the *subnucleus reticularis dorsalis* (SRD) in nociception. The reciprocal connections between the SRD and spinal cord suggest that this area is an important link in feedback loops which regulate spinal outflow. Moreover, the existence of SRD-thalamic connections cast new light on the role of spino-reticulo-thalamo-cortical circuits in pain processing

thalamic nociceptive branch of what was originally termed the "ascending reticular activating system" [44-47].

Moreover, the cortical layer I areas that receive the densest efferent projections from the VM thalamus also contain the greatest number of neurones in cortical layers V-VI that project to the VM*l* and SRD [41, 48].

Conclusions

Modifications in the activity of large groups of thalamo-cortical cells have been associated with changes in states of consciousness [49]. This hypothesis is in accordance with the fact that painful stimuli can elicit widespread cortical activation [50, 51]. It is further supported by studies using calibrated painful stimuli in humans which have demonstrated not only the activation of various areas of cortex but also with increasing stimulus intensity, of an increasing number of regions of the brain [52]. Interestingly, some areas such as the ventral posterior and medial thalamic regions and the prefrontal, premotor and motor cortices showed significant increases in activity bilaterally [52].

It is tempting to speculate that the SRD-thalamo-cortical network may allow painful stimuli to modify cortical activity in a universal way. The VM thalamus-cortical reciprocal connections could feedback inputs which may engage other, adjacent, areas of the cortex and so disperse activity in a widespread fashion. From a general point of view, our data support hypotheses implicating large groups of thalamic neurones as potential relays for controlling behavioural levels of attention and/or for the planning of programmed movements [47, 53, 54].

Acknowledgements. The authors are grateful to some members of the U-161 for their contribution to some aspects of this work. This work was supported by l'Institut National de la Santé et de la Recherche Médicale (INSERM) and l'Institut UPSA de la douleur.

References

1. Mehler WR, Feferman ME, Nauta WJH (1960) Ascending axon degeneration following antero-lateral corodotomy, an experimental study in the monkey. Brain 83:718-751
2. Bowsher D (1957) Termination of the central pain pathway in man: the conscious appreciation of pain. Brain 80:606-622
3. Bowsher D (1962) The topographical projection of fibres from the anterolateral quadrant of the spinal cord to the subdiencephalic brain stem in man. Psychiatr Neurol 143:75-99
4. Kohnstamm O, Quensel F (1908) Das centrum receptorium (sensorium) der formatio reticularis. Neurol Zbl 27:1046-1047
5. Quensel F (1907) Präparate mit aktiven Zelldegenerationen nach Hirnstammverletzung bei Kaninchen. Neurol Zbl 26:1138-1139
6. Bowsher D (1976) Role of the reticular formation in responses to noxious stimulation. Pain 2:361-378
7. Gebhart GF (1982) Opiate and opioid peptide effects on brain stem neurons: relevance to nociception and antinociceptive mechanisms. Pain 12:93-140
8. Villanueva L, Bouhassira D, Le Bars D (1996) The medullary subnucleus reticularis dorsalis (SRD) as a key link in both the transmission and modulation of pain signals. Pain 67:231-240
9. Casey KL (1969) Somatosensory responses of bulboreticular units in the awake cat: relation to escape producing stimuli. Science 173:77-80
10. Casey KL (1971) Escape elicited by bulboreticular stimulation in the cat. Int J Neurosci 2:29-34

11. Valverde F (1961) Reticular formation of the pons and medulla oblongata. A Golgi study. J Comp Neurol 116:71-99
12. Valverde F (1962) Reticular formation of the albino rat's brainstem: cytoarchitecture and corticofugal connections. J Comp Neurol 119:25-49
13. Newman DB (1985) Distinguishing rat brainstem reticulospinal nuclei by their neuronal morphology. I. Medullary nuclei. J Hirnforsch 26:187-226
14. Villanueva L, Bouhassira D, Bing Z, Le Bars D (1988) Convergence of heterotopic nociceptive information onto subnucleus reticularis dorsalis neurons in the rat medulla. J Neurophysiol 60:980-1009
15. Villanueva L, Bing Z, Le Bars D (1994) Effects of heterotopic noxious stimuli on activity of neurones in Subnucleus Reticularis Dorsalis in the rat medulla. J Physiol (London) 475:255-266
16. Villanueva L, Bing Z, Bouhassira D, Le Bars D (1989) Encoding of electrical, thermal and mechanical noxious stimuli by subnucleus reticularis dorsalis neurons in the rat medulla. J Neurophysiol 61:391-402
17. Roy JC, Bing Z, Villanueva L, Le Bars D (1992) Convergence of visceral and somatic inputs onto subnucleus reticularis dorsalis neurones in the rat medulla. J Physiol (London) 452:235-246
18. Villanueva L, Cliffer KD, Sorkin L et al (1990) Convergence of heterotopic nociceptive information onto neurons of the caudal medullary reticular formation in the monkey (Macaca fascicularis). J Neurophysiol 63:1118-1127
19. Bing Z, Villanueva L, Le Bars D (1990) Ascending pathways in the spinal cord involved in the activation of subnucleus reticularis dorsalis neurons in the medulla of the rat. J Neurophysiol 63:424-438
20. Villanueva L, Nathan PW (2000) Multiple pain pathways. In: Devor M, Rowbotham, MC, Wiesendfeld-Hallin Z (eds) Proceedings of the Ninth World Congress on Pain. IASP, Seattle, pp 371-386
21. Lima D (1990) A spinomedullary projection terminating in the dorsal reticular nucleus of the rat. Neuroscience 34:577-590
22. Villanueva L, De Pommery J, Menétrey D, Le Bars D (1991) Spinal afferent projections to subnucleus reticularis dorsalis in the rat. Neurosci Lett 134:98-102
23. Yezierski RP, Broton JG (1991) Functional properties of spino-mesencephalic tract (SMT) cells in the upper cervical spinal cord of the cat. Pain 45:187-196
24. Smith MV, Apkarian AV, Hodge CJ (1991) Somatosensory response properties of contralaterally projecting spinothalamic and non-spinothalamic neurons in the second cervical segment of the cat. J Neurophysiol 66:83-102
25. Willis WD, Coggeshall RE (1991) Sensory mechanisms of the spinal cord. Plenum, New York
26. Hitchcock E (1970) Stereotaxic cervical myelotomy. J Neurol Neurosurg Psychiatry 33:224-230
27. Papo I, Luongo A (1976) High cervical commissural myelotomy in the treatment of pain. J Neurol Neurosurg Psychiatry 39:705-710
28. Schvarcz JR (1977) Functional exploration of the spinomedullary junction. Acta Neurochir Suppl (Wien) 24:179-185
29. Sourek K (1977) Mediolongitudinal myelotomy. Prog Neurol Surg 8:15-34
30. Cook AW, Nathan PW, Smith MC (1984) Sensory consequences of commissural myelotomy. A challenge to traditional anatomical concepts. Brain 107:547-568
31. Villanueva L, Bernard JF, Le Bars D (1995) Distribution of spinal cord projections from the medullary subnucleus reticularis dorsalis and the adjacent cuneate nucleus: a phaseolus vulgaris leucoagglutinin (PHA-L) study in the rat. J Comp Neurol 352:11-32

32. Raboisson P, Dallel R, Bernard JF et al (1996) Organization of efferent projections from the spinal cervical enlargement to the medullary subnucleus reticularis dorsalis and the adjacent cuneate nucleus: a PHA-L study in the rat. J Comp Neurol 367:503-517
33. Almeida A, Tavares I, Lima D, Coimbra A (1993) Descending projections from the medullary dorsal reticular nucleus make synaptic contacts with spinal cord lamina I cells projecting to that nucleus: an electron microscopic tracer study in the rat. Neuroscience 55:1093-1106
34. Almeida A, Tavares I, Lima D (2000) Reciprocal connections between the medullary dorsal reticular nucleus and the spinal dorsal horn in the rat (Submitted)
35. Villanueva L, Le Bars D (1995) The activation of bulbo-spinal controls by peripheral nociceptive inputs: diffuse noxious inhibitory controls (DNIC). Biol Res 28:113-125
36. Bing Z, Villanueva L, Le Bars D (1990) Acupuncture and diffuse noxious inhibitory controls: naloxone reversible depression of activities of trigeminal convergent neurones. Neuroscience 37:809-818
37. Bouhassira D, Villanueva L, Bing Z, Le Bars D (1992) Involvement of the subnucleus reticularis dorsalis in diffuse noxious inhibitory controls in the rat. Brain Res 595:353-357
38. De Broucker T, Cesaro P, Willer JC, Le Bars D (1990) Diffuse noxious inhibitory controls (DNIC) in man: involvement of a spino-reticular tract. Brain 113:1223-1234
39. Villanueva L, Desbois C, Le Bars D, Bernard JF (1998) Organization of diencephalic projections from the medullary subnucleus reticularis dorsalis and the adjacent cuneate nucleus: a retrograde and anterograde tracer study in the rat. J Comp Neurol 390:133-160
40. Monconduit L, Bourgeais L, Bernard JF et al (1999) Ventromedial thalamic neurons convey nociceptive signals from the whole body surface to the dorsolateral neocortex. J Neurosci 19:9063-9072
41. Desbois C, Villanueva L (2000) The organization of lateral ventromedial thalamic connections in the rat: a link for the distribution of nociceptive signals to widespread cortical regions (Submitted)
42. Cajal SR (1972) Histologie du Système Nerveux de l'Homme et des Vertébrés [Reprinted from the original (1911)]. Maloine, Paris
43. Marín-Padilla M (1998) Cajal-Retzius cells and the development of the neocortex. Trends Neurosci 21:64-71
44. Morison RS, Dempsey EW (1942) A study of thalamo-cortical relations. Am J Physiol 135: 281-292
45. Moruzzi G, Magoun HW (1949) Brain stem reticular formation and activation of the EEG. Electroencephalogr Clin Neurophysiol 1:445-473
46. Jasper HH (1961) Thalamic reticular system. In: Sheer DE (ed) Electrical stimulation of the brain. Austin University Press, Austin, pp 277-287
47. Herkenham M (1986) New perspectives on the organization and evolution of nonspecific thalamocortical projections. In: Jones EG, Peters A (eds) Sensory-motor areas and aspects of cortical connectivity. Plenum, New York, pp 403-445 (Cerebral cortex, vol. 5)
48. Desbois C, Le Bars D, Villanueva L (1999) Organization of cortical projections to the medullary subnucleus reticularis dorsalis: a retrograde and anterograde tracing study in the rat. J Comp Neurol 410:178-196
49. Steriade M, Contreras D, Amzica F (1997) The thalamocortical dialogue during wake, sleep and paroxysmal oscillations. In: Steriade M, Jones EG, McCormick DA (eds) Thalamus. Elsevier, Amsterdam, pp 213-294
50. Porro CA, Cavazzuti M (1996) Functional imaging studies of the pain system in man and animals. In: Carli G, Zimmerman M (eds) Towards the neurobiology of chronic pain. Elsevier, New York, pp 47-62 (Progress in brain research, vol. 110)

51. Treede RD, Kenshalo DR, Gracely RH, Jones AK (1999) The cortical representation of pain. Pain 79:105-111
52. Derbyshire SW, Jones AK, Gyulai F et al (1997) Pain processing during three levels of noxious stimulation produces differential patterns of central activity. Pain 73:431-445
53. Groenewegen HJ, Berendse HW (1994) The specificity of the 'nonspecific' midline and intralaminar thalamic nuclei. Trends Neurosci 17:52-57
54. Jones EG (1998) Viewpoint: the core and matrix of thalamic organization. Neuroscience 85:331-345
55. Paxinos G, Watson C (1997) The rat brain in stereotaxic coordinates. Academic, New York

Chapter 5

The Thalamus and Pain

M.L. Sotgiu

The thalamus is the relay for the transmission of information on all sensory modalities to the cortex and is considered a key for the receipt, integration and transfer of nociceptive information, also displaying an important modulatory role. The thalamus encodes information about the type, temporal pattern, intensity, and, at least for cutaneous input, topographic localization of pain. It interacts with cortical and limbic structures responsible for both the sensory-discriminative and emotional dimensions of pain.

In the last few years significant advances have been made in the understanding of thalamic involvement in the mechanisms of nociception with electrophysiological and neuroimaging techniques. Particular interest has been put on the following points: the discharge properties of the thalamic neurons during processing of nociceptive information, taking into account the bi-directional circuits that interconnect the thalamus and the cortex with reciprocal modulation of their activity; the interaction of neuronal activity with neurotransmitter systems; the behavior of thalamic structures during the different pain states; and the relationship between the functional reorganization after peripheral or central lesion and the pain.

The results indicate that, besides some common basis for the acute and chronic pain signals (pathways of transmission, neurotransmitters, kind of neurons), different adaptive events occur in chronic pain states.

Basically, the nociceptive inputs from the spinal cord to the thalamus are conveyed through the spinothalamic tract (STT) and in part through the spinoreticulothalamic tract (SRTT). The terminations are distributed throughout the medial and the lateral thalamus with a STT dense projection in the ventroposterior lateral (VPL), ventroposterior medial (VPM), ventroposterior inferior (VPI), and posterior (PO) nuclei of the lateral thalamus, and in the intralaminar and submedius nuclei of the medial thalamus.

The thalamic neurons, both the thalamocortical relay neurons that transmit information to the cortex and the GABAergic interneurons devoted to local inhibition, function in two basic modes: the relay mode, characterized by constant firing rate, and the oscillatory mode, characterized by high frequency bursts of action potentials preceded by prolonged decreases in the firing rate. Through the relay mode, the thalamic neurons faithfully transmit afferent signals to the cortex.

An important role in the modulation of inputs relayed by the thalamic nuclei is played by the nucleus reticularis thalamus (RT), a sheet-like field surrounding the rostrolateral surfaces of the thalamic mass composed by inhibitory neurons (GABAergic neurons). RT has reciprocal interconnections with the thalamic nuclei and is a relay for the descending corticothalamic connection that, through the activation of the RT neurons, exert its inhibitory action on the thalamic transmission of the signals [1].

The Thalamus and Chronic Pain

The nociceptive information is processed differently in acute and chronic pain. Indeed, the mechanisms subserving the signaling of acute pain induced, for example, by a brief noxious stimulus, can be viewed as a fairly simple route of transmission centrally toward the thalamus and the cortex and thus the consciousness, with possible modulation at synaptic relays along the way. By contrast chronic pain is underlined by substantial alterations in the normal nociceptive system; it is maintained by anomalous activity at all the relays of the central nervous system (CNS), which may be internally generated or driven by abnormal peripheral inputs.

Alterations in neuronal responsiveness and reorganization of patterns of synaptic connectivity occur along the entire transmission pathway, from the spinal cord to the cortex. At the thalamic relay the neuronal activity may reflect a balance of influences involving both bottom-up and top-down processes.

This article focuses on the thalamus and chronic pain (neurogenic pain), in an attempt to describe the mechanisms underlying the states of central hypersensitization and of increased signal transmission by which pain is transformed from a transient sensation to a persistent disorder.

The chronic neurogenic pain is produced by lesions along the somatosensory pathways from the peripheral nerve to the cortex. As widely documented in the humans and in the animal models of pain, it is generally correlated to an abnormal neuronal excitability at the various levels of the somatosensorial system, joined to a complex reorganization of the central representation of the projection fields and to changes in the receptorial system of the neuro-transmitters.

The most important changes that intervene in the thalamic regions include:
1. Modifications in the pattern discharges and in the discharge frequency of the thalamic neurons.
2. Modification in the inhibition-excitation equilibrium through a decreased level of GABA.
3. Functional and/or anatomical reorganization.

Changes in Neuronal Activity

One main finding is that the neuronal thalamic activity not only may change the discharge frequency but also, maintaining the same frequency, the pattern discharge. This means that the change in the characteristic pattern of discharges could not involve modifications in firing frequency.

Furthermore, the discharge of the thalamic neurons may shift from the single spike or relay mode to abnormal bursting or oscillatory mode [2].

The mechanisms involved in these kinds of activity have been clarified by intracellular studies. The relay mode is related to a membrane depolarization with respect to the resting potential. The depolarization through a slowly inactivating sodium conductance induces a continuous depolarizing current that, in turn, activates a sodium action potential, followed by an afterhyperpolarization that produces a refractory period. This sequence results in the constant firing rate characteristic of the relay mode.

The bursting or oscillatory mode is related to a membrane hyperpolarization with respect to the resting potential. In this case, the inhibitory postsynaptic potentials (IPSPs) may be prolonged and during the recovery of the resting potential there is an increase in calcium conductance that provides a low-threshold, rapidly inactivating calcium current. This sequence results in a series of action potentials at high frequency, termed low-threshold calcium-spike-associated burst.

In studies on the thalamic neuronal activity after spinal cord injury, a more frequent occurrence of bursting of the type associated with calcium spikes was found in patients with pain than in patients without pain [3, 4], indicating that this phenomenon may be related to the sensation of pain. Furthermore, the generation of low-threshold calcium spike (LTS) bursts by thalamic neurons seems to be involved in the thalamocortical dysrhythmia, a phenomenon observed in patients suffering from neurogenic pain [5]. Thus, some types of pain may be represented by a disorder of normal thalamic discharging mechanisms rather than by a quantitative variation in frequency discharge.

On the other hand, in experimental animal models of neuropathic pain, Biella [6] describes characteristic dynamics of discharges of thalamocortical neurons in which an increased frequency and a loss of spatiotemporal organization of the inputs induce a perturbation of the circuits. The disorganized input from the ascending spinal pathways [7] can partially account for those disorders. The increased mean frequency of discharge of the thalamic VPL neurons is characterized by disordered patterns, with sudden switches from tonic hyperactivity to bursting activity and back. Single neurons present stable discharge anomalies: these can be due both to the disordered input patterns and to the changed electrochemical properties of the units due to the imported pathological conditions. Examples from the spinal cord sensory neurons have, in fact, shown that new genes sets are unveiled in the pathological conditions in the periphery, Fos, Jun and Krox-24 being the ones studied most. New ionic channel protein genes have also been described, the latter inducing fatal changes to the electrochemical properties of the cells. Some inferences about the new channel configuration can be drawn from processing data on neural networks but this issue will not be discussed further in this context. These disordered activities, read at the level of units, also influence the network behavior. The strong functional relationships between these complex structures imply that the mutual dependence of neurons also relies on local changes. Where the thalamus is involved by the neuronal activity change, the cortical circuits are involved too. In the rat this tenet is even stronger in that there are no clear excitatory connections among relay cells by recurrent collaterals. Under experimental conditions, the rats with a peripheral mononeuropathy show a strongly decreased index of correlation among the cells despite the increased overall discharge frequency. The apparent paradox could be due to a decrease in correct timing windows used for thalamocortical functional connectivity. The unbalanced external input activations should disrupt the normal thalamocortical loop. The disruption of the timed reverberation leads to a decrease in network cell entrainment and to the independence of single units. The network tends to loosen the inner connectivity and to decrease the estimation of both external and internal inputs, the input estimates being worked out as a distributed process.

Inhibitory System

Under normal condition a model of intrathalamic connectivity has been proposed in which the organization of sensory transmission is regulated by inhibitory neurons that use the transmitter GABA [8].

Damage in the sensory pathway may disrupt the normal dynamic state of equilibrium between excitation and inhibition within the network that comprises the entire somatosensory system, with a decreased level of GABA. This results in a reduced inhibition of transmission neurons with a consequent neuronal hyperexcitability or hyperactivity and thus also in the amplification of the signals.

Furthermore, a reduction in GABAergic tone inducing neuronal disinhibition may set off reverberatory firing patterns in nociceptive circuits.

Many data in the literature indicate that the GABAergic inhibitory neurons are crucial for controlling (negatively) the nociceptive processes in the thalamic relay neurons and support the notion that the disruption of GABAergic transmission in the thalamus, disinhibiting the transfer of nociceptive information, contributes to painful states.

Reorganization

The reorganization of the central representation of peripheral fields has been widely studied in human and in experimental animals with acute, reversible or chronic deafferentation. In all cases, expansion of somatotopically adjacent regions into deafferented areas has been described.

In humans who had suffered spinal transections at various levels, an expanded representation of the juxta-anesthetic region has been described [4]. Furthermore, microstimulation studies in patients with pain due to nervous system injury indicate that the reorganization may concern not only the thalamic maps but also the sensory modalities that change, for example, from thermal to noxious [9]. It is evident that in such cases the modality plasticity may contribute to the development of chronic pain.

Furthermore, other than the somatotopic reorganization, it is suggested that there is a redistribution of function in the somatosensory pathway through extensive plastic reorganization [10] so that functions usually performed by one region may be taken over by another. It is known, in fact, that central lesions induce anatomical deafferentations of the thalamus whereas a peripheral lesion produces only its functional deafferentation [11].

In conclusion, the changes here described contribute to the amplification of the nociceptive signals, to the extension of areas of transmission of nociceptive information, and to the maintenance of these altered functions of the nociceptive system at the thalamic level.

Neuroimaging

Imaging studies of the activation of the thalamus were performed with positron emission tomography (PET), single photon emission tomography (SPET), and functional magnetic resonance imaging (fMRI) techniques, to obtain additional information about the involvement of this area in pain. The more consistent results were obtained in studies on acute pain in healthy volunteers and reveal significant increases in activity in the thalamus contralateral to the noxious stimulation [12].

Less consistent are the results concerning the behavior of thalamic activity in chronic pain states. Indeed, in PET studies, a decrease in contralateral thalamic activity was found in patients with chronic pain due to cancer [13], in patients with chronic neuropathic pain [14] and in patients with chronic pain due to nervous lesions not involving gangliar function [15], no changes in the thalamic activity in patients with chronic neuropathic pain [16] and in patients with chronic pain due to nervous lesion involving ganglionic function [15]. On the other hand, in a SPECT study in patients with central post-stroke pain, an increase in thalamic activity was found only in those with clinical signs of hyperpathia and not in patients without hyperpathia [17].

To explain these contrasting results three main scenarios could be hypothesized:
1. A strong barrage of nociceptive inputs can inhibit the afferences conveying other modalities (the thalamic interconnections are suitable for this mechanism): this behavior may result in a reduction of total thalamic activity.
2. Central post stroke pain is associated with sensorial disturbances so that the thalamus also processes other sensorial modalities as nociceptive: this behavior may result in an increase in total thalamic activity.
3. Central pain of different origin that in its initial phase, seems underlined by thalamic hyperactivity, as widely shown in animal models [18] is sustained by a stabilized thalamic activity after a variable period of time. A new equilibrium inhibition-excitation can be organized if there are degenerations of excitatory and/or inhibitory pathways. No changes of activity would result in this condition.

From the neuroimaging data it is clear that not all kinds of chronic pain have an evident correlate in the change of thalamic activity and that several variables must be considered as contributing to the different results.

One variable may be the kind of injury underlying the chronic pain, in particular whether the damage implies degenerative processes or not. Another variable may relate alterations in the thalamic activity to microvascular deficit. Another important, although not quantifiable, factor to be taken into consideration is that a characteristic of chronic neurogenic pain in humans is the influence of emotional factors. The direct thalamocortical and corticothalamic connections of all mesocortical areas provide the anatomical basis for the emotional influence. It seems to be related to the different conditions: an intact thalamus or a thalamus that undergoes functional vs anatomical reorganization after central or peripheral damage.

References

1. Jones EG (1990) The thalamus. Plenum, New York
2. Steriade M, Jones EG, Llinas RR (1990) Thalamic oscillations and signaling. Wiley, New York
3. Lenz FA, Kwan HC, Dostrovsky JO, Tasker RR (1989) Characteristics of the bursting pattern of action potentials that occurs in the thalamus of patients with central pain. Brain Res 496:357-360
4. Lenz FA, Kwan HC, Martin R et al (1994) Characteristics of somatotopic organization and spontaneous neuronal activity in the region of the thalamic principal sensory nucleus in patients with spinal cord transection. J Neurophysiol 72:1570-1587
5. Llinas RR, Ribary U, Jeanmonod D et al (1999) Thalamocortical dysrhythmia: a neurological and neuropsychiatric syndrome characterized by magnetoencephalography. Proc Natl Acad Sci USA 96:15222-15227
6. Biella G (2000) Thalamo-cortical neuronal firing coincidence disorders in animal model of neuropathic pain (in prep)
7. Biella G, Riva L, Sotgiu ML (1997) Interaction between neurons in different laminae of the dorsal horn of the spinal cord. A correlation study in normal and neuropathic rats. Eur J Neurosci 9:1017-1025
8. Roberts WA, Eaton SA, Salt TE (1992) Widely distributed GABA-mediated afferent inhibition processes within the ventrobasal thalamus of rat and their possible relevance to pathological pain states and somatotopic plasticity. Exp Brain Res 89:363-372
9. Lenz FA, Gracely RH, Baker FH et al (1998) Reorganization of sensory modalities evoked by microstimulation in region of the thalamic principal sensory nucleus in patients with pain due to nervous system injury. J Comp Neurol 399:125-138
10. Garraghty PE, Kaas JE (1991) Functional reorganization in adult monkey thalamus after a peripheral nerve injury. NeuroReport 2:747-750
11. Janmonod D, Magin M, Morel A (1993) Thalamus and neurogenic pain: physiological, anatomical and clinical data. NeuroReport 4:474-478
12. Casey KL (1999) Blochade forebrain mechanisms of nociception and pain: analysis though imaging. Proc Natl Acad Sci USA 96:7668-7674
13. Di Piero V, Jones AKP, Jannotti F et al (1991) Chronic pain: a PET study of the central effects of percutaneous high cervical cordotomy. Pain 46:9-12
14. Iadarola MJ, Max M B, Berman KF et al (1995) Unilateral decrease in thalamic activity observed with positron emission tomography in patients with chronic neuropathic pain. Pain 63:55-64
15. Marchettini P, Sotgiu ML, Lucignani G et al (1995) Chronic pain and thalamic activity studied by PET. EFIC Abst. 149
16. Hsieh JC, Belfrage M, Stone-Elander S et al (1995) Central representation of chronic ongoing neuropathic pain studied by positron emission tomography. Pain 63:225-236
17. Cesaro P, Mann MW, Moretti JL et al (1991) Central pain and thalamic hyperactivity: a single photon emission computerized tomographic study. Pain 47:329-336
18. Guilbaud G, Benoist JM, Jazat F, Gautron M (1990) Neuronal responsiveness in the ventrobasal thalamic complex of rats with an experimental peripheral mononeuropathy. J Neurophysiol 64:1537-1554

Chapter 6

Naloxone, but not Estradiol, Affects the Gonadectomy-Induced Increase in Hippocampal Cholineacetyltransferase Activity in Male Rats

I. Ceccarelli, A. Scaramuzzino, A.M. Aloisi

Cholinergic neurons located in the medial septum and the diagonal band of Broca are a major source of cholinergic innervation to the hippocampal formation. These neurons play an important role in learning and memory processes [1]. Gonadal hormones can significantly affect the function of these cholinergic neurons [2]. Estrogens were found to increase cholineacetyltransferase (ChAT) activity and the number of ChAT neurons in the medial septum in ovariectomized female rats [3]. Moreover, estrogens significantly improve cognition capacities in menopausal women treated with estrogen-replacement therapy [4]. Although not a limiting factor in the synthesis of ACh, ChAT activity is considered an index of cholinergic activation [5]. We have previously shown that a persistent, painful stimulus (formalin test) decreases ChAT activity in male rats, an effect not present in females [6], and induces higher c-Fos expression levels in the hippocampus of female rats than in males [7].

The principal male gonadal hormone, testosterone, acts in the CNS through androgen receptors (AR). It also exerts important actions through its products, DHT (after hydrogenation) and estradiol (after aromatization). An important link between estradiol and pain is the hormone's ability to modulate the opioid system. Indeed, the modulation by estrogens of the synthesis and secretion of β-EP in the hypothalamic arcuate nucleus of female rats is well known [8].

The present study was designed to determine the effects of gonadal hormone depletion on hippocampal ChAT activity and the short-term effects of estradiol administration in pain-free and formalin-treated male rats. Naloxone was administered to determine whether the effects were mediated by opioid substances. All the treatments were administered intracerebrocircularly (icv) in order to act specifically on supraspinal central receptors.

Materials and Methods

Subjects

The subjects were 65 male Wistar rats (Harlan-Nossan, Italy), weighing 220-240 g upon arrival. All experimental procedures followed the regulations of the European Communities Council Directive 86/609/EEC and the ethical guidelines for the study of experimental pain in conscious animals [9]. The rats were kept on a 12-h dark/light cycle, with the dark phase occurring during daylight hours. While in the home cage, the rats were allowed ad libitum access to food and water.

Surgery

Under pentobarbital anesthesia (40 mg/kg, i.p.), half of the animals were gonadectomized (GDX), while in the other animals the testes were only exposed (Intact). Two weeks later, anesthesia was repeated in all animals and a guide cannula (22-gauge, 15 mm) equipped with a 28-gauge stylet was implanted in the third ventricle (AP = -1.4, L = 1.4, H = -3.4 mm). The cannula was attached to the skull with a stainless steel screw and acrylic cement. The animals were left to recover for 7-10 days before the behavioral testing.

Experimental Design

Twenty-one days after gonadectomy or sham surgery, the GDX and Intact rats were randomly assigned to one of four experimental groups, depending on the administration of saline or 17β-estradiol (1 µg/5 µl, icv) on the 2 days before the formalin test and on the administration of saline or naloxone (2,5 µg/5 µl, icv) 15 min before the formalin test: (1) group SAL1/SAL2, which received only an icv injection of saline on days 20, 21 and 22 ($n = 10$ GDX and $n = 11$ Intact); (2) group SAL1/NAL, which received saline on days 20 and 21 and naloxone on day 22 ($n = 10$ GDX and $n = 12$ Intact); (3) ESTR/SAL2, which received estradiol on days 20 and 21 and saline on days 22 ($n = 11$ GDX and $n = 13$ Intact); and (4) ESTR/NAL, which received estradiol on days 20 and 21 and naloxone on days 22 ($n = 1$ GDX and $n = 12$ Intact). For each experimental group, half of the animals ($n = 5$-7) were randomly assigned to the formalin-treated (FORM) groups and half ($n = 5$-7) to the sham-treated (SHAM) groups. On the day of the experiment, animals were transported singly to the testing room, which was supplied with red light and in which the temperature was maintained at the same level as the animal house (24 ± 1°C).

All icv injections were given in a 5-µl volume which was infused (Hamilton syringe and polyethylene tubing) at a rate of 1 µl every 5-6 s. β-Estradiol-water soluble (Sigma Chemical, St. Louis, USA) and naloxone hydrochloride (Sigma Chemical) were dissolved in 0,9% saline for the icv injections. We performed icv injections by gently restraining the rat, removing the stylet and inserting the injection cannula; a total volume of 5 µl was infused (Hamilton syringe and polyethylene tube) over a 30-s period. Twenty seconds after the drugs were infused, the injector was removed and replaced with the stylet and the animal was returned to its home cage. Fifteen minutes after the injection of naloxone/saline, the animal was again gently restrained. If it belonged to the FORM group, it received a subcutaneous injection of formalin (5%, 50 µl) in the dorsal part of the hind paw, while if part of the SHAM group, it received only a needle prick, i.e., it was exposed to the same physical stimuli but not to the subcutaneous injection of a substance. Immediately thereafter, the animal was placed in a novel behavioral apparatus made of transparent Plexiglas (50 x 50 x 30 cm high), with lines painted on the floor to form 25 equal squares. The apparatus was equipped with an infrared video camera so that the animal's behavior could be recorded in another room. The apparatus was carefully cleaned with water after the testing of each animal. All testing took place between 10 and 14 h during the dark phase, i.e., the activity period of the rats, to avoid interference of the experimental procedures with sleep.

At the end of the formalin test, all animals were killed by decapitation and blood was collected from the trunk in EDTA-added beakers for testosterone determination. The brain was removed and checked for appropriate placement of the cannula. The two hippocampi were dissected and immediately frozen (−20°C) for subsequent ChAT activity determination.

Hormonal assays

Testosterone plasma levels were determined by radioimmunoassay as previously described [10].

ChAT determination

ChAT activity was determined according to the Fonnum radiochemical method [11], with slight modifications, and expressed as micromoles of ACh/h per 100 mg of proteins.

Analysis of variance (ANOVA) was applied to ChAT activity values and hormone levels with the factors gonadectomy (two levels: Intact, GDX), estrogen (two levels: SAL1, ESTR), naloxone (two levels: SAL2, NAL) and formalin (two levels: Sham, Form). The LSD test was used for post-hoc comparisons when needed. Pearson's Linear Correlation test was applied to ChAT activity and testosterone plasma levels.

Results

ANOVA applied to ChAT activity revealed a significant effect of the factors gonadectomy [$F(1.49) = 64,63$; $p < 0,001$] and Naloxone [$F(1.49) = 4,56, p < 0,03$] and a significant interaction gonadectomy × naloxone [$F(1.49) = 5,81, p < 0,02$]. As shown in Figure 1, this was due to the higher levels of ChAT activity in GDX animals than in Intact ones. Moreover, the increase was not present in GDX animals pre-treated with naloxone.

Estrogen treatment resulted in a slight increase in ChAT activity which did not reach significance, particularly not in sham-treated animals. In all cases, naloxone pre-treatment abolished these effects. The subcutaneous injection of formalin did not induce any significant changes in ChAT activity, neither in Intact animals nor in GDX ones.

Gonadectomy drastically reduced testosterone plasma levels in all animals, as shown by the significance of the factor gonadectomy [$F(1.65) = 66,1, p < 0,001$] due to the lower levels in GDX animals than intact ones. In addition, the significance of the interaction gonadectomy × estrogen [$F(1.65) = 6.7, p < 0.01$] was due to the

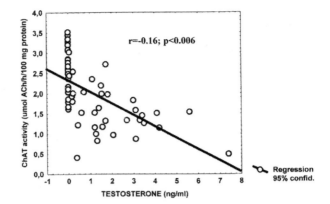

Fig. 1. Hippocampal ChAT activity determined in Intact and GDX male rats subjected to the formalin test: sham-treatment or formalin-treatment (50 μl, 5%). SAL1/SAL2 rats received saline for 2 days (*SAL1*) and then again 15 min before the formalin test (*SAL2*); SAL1/NAL rats received saline for 2 days (*SAL1*) and naloxone 15 min before the formalin test (*NAL*); ESTR/SAL2 rats received estrogen for 2 days (*ESTR*) and saline 15 min before the formalin test (*SAL2*); ESTR/NAL rats received estrogen for 2 days (*ESTR*) and naloxone 15 min before the formalin test (*NAL*)

estrogen-induced decrease of testosterone levels in Intact animals but not in GDX ones (Fig. 2).

There was a negative correlation between testosterone plasma levels and ChAT activity in the hippocampus ($n = 58$; r = $-0,61, p < 001$) (Fig. 3).

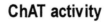

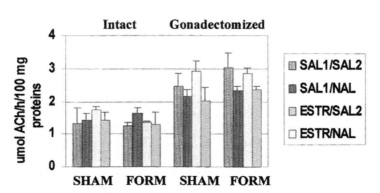

Fig. 2. Testosterone plasma levels. Groups as in Figure 1. Note the different *scale bar* between Intact and GDX animals

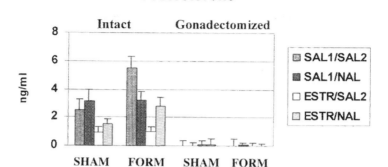

Fig 3. Linear correlation between testosterone plasma levels and ChAT activity ($N = 58$)

Discussion

The present study clearly demonstrates that testosterone in male rats acts on the septohippocampal cholinergic neurons to depress hippocampal ChAT activity. Indeed, 3 weeks after gonadectomy, GDX male rats showed higher ChAT activity than intact males, suggesting a loss of an inhibitory effect of testosterone.

Luine and co-workers have reported that estrogen replacement administration in adult ovariectomized (OVX) female rats can result in increased ChAT activity in the hippocampus [12]. More recently, Gibbs et al. found that 2 days of s.c. estrogen treatment were enough to increase ChAT mRNA in the hippocampus of OVX female rats [13]. In the present experiment, gonadectomy induced an increase instead of a decrease in ChAT activity. Interestingly, this increase is in agreement with the observations in rodents of an inhibitory role of testosterone in other CNS structures, as well as with reports showing that testosterone administration is not able to restore the age-dependent ChAT activity decrease [14]. Moreover, Pan et al. [15] recently showed that both estradiol and soy phytoestrogens do not affect ChAT mRNA levels in the frontal cortex and hippocampus of young OVX female rats.

It is important to underline the fact that the ChAT activity determined in the present experiment was the result of dynamic processes occurring during the formalin test (60 min). During this test, the animals were exposed to a novel environment and, if treated with formalin, experienced a persistent, painful stimulus. Thus, although gonadectomy occurred 3 weeks before the behavioral test, the septo-hippocampal cholinergic system was strongly modulated by the exposure to these stimuli; this has repeatedly been shown with the microdialysis technique, by which it is possible to directly measure the ACh released by the septohippocampal cholinergic terminals [16]. The inverse relationship between ChAT activity and testosterone levels strongly supports this hypothesis. Since this effect was not restored by estradiol administration, it must be considered an effect directly mediated by testosterone or by other testosterone-related products but not by the estradiol which can be obtained after aromatization.

On the whole, it appears that testosterone acts in the hippocampal neurons to keep the activity of the cholinergic system at low levels. This inhibitory effect is lost after gonadectomy.

Interestingly, this inhibitory effect seems to be restored by the icv injection of naloxone. The ability of naloxone to interfere with GDX-induced increases of ChAT activity suggests a direct modulation by opioids of testosterone-sensitive neurons. Already in 1978, Moroni [17] showed the ability of endorphin to modulate cholinergic neurons. ACh release usually appears to be depressed by β-EP, but the data are not unequivocal. Opioids seem to act in the hippocampus through opioid receptors (repeatedly described in the hippocampal subfields), but also through the receptors present in the medial septum (including opioid receptors). Vernadokis and Kentroti [18] showed in vitro that cultures treated with anti-met-enkephalin antiserum or naloxone exhibited a neuronal growth pattern different from that of controls.

In the present experiment it is important to emphasize that the effects are independent of the presence of a persistent nociceptive input. This implies that the opiadergic system involved in cholinergic modulation is different from that involved in pain mechanisms.

In conclusion, gonadal hormones seem to greatly affect hippocampal functions also in males, and with different neuronal effects from those observed in females. Further studies are needed to identify more clearly the neuronal circuits involved.

Acknowledgements. This work was supported by MURST and University of Siena funds.

References

1. Dutar P, Bassant MH, Senut MC, Lamour Y (1995) The septohippocampal pathway: structure and function of a central cholinergic system. Physiol Rev 75:393-427
2. Luine VN (1997) Steroid hormone modulation of hippocampal dependent spatial memory. Stress 2:21-36
3. Gibbs RB, Pfaff DW (1992) Effects of estrogen and fimbria/fornix transection on p75NGFR and ChAT expression in the medial septum and diagonal band of Broca. Exp Neurol 116:23-39
4. Paganini-Hill A, Henderson VW (1996) Estrogen replacement therapy and risk of Alzheimer disease. Arch Intern Med 156:2213-2217
5. Schmidt BM, Rylett RJ (1993) Phosphorylation of rat brain choline acetyltransferase and its relationship to enzyme activity. J Neurochem 61:1774-1781
6. Aloisi AM, Albonetti ME, Carli G (1996) Formalin-induced changes in adrenocorticotropic hormone and corticosterone plasma levels and hippocampal choline acetyltransferase activity in male and female rats. Neuroscience 74:1019-1024
7. Aloisi AM, Zimmermann M, Herdegen T (1997) Sex-dependent effects of formalin and restraint on c-Fos expression in the septum and hippocampus of the rat. Neuroscience 81:951-958
8. Toran-Allerand CD, Singh M, Setalo G Jr (1990) Novel mechanisms of estrogen action in the brain: new players in an old story. Front Neuroendocrinol 20:97-121

9. Zimmermann M (1983) Ethical guidelines for investigations of experimental pain in conscious animals. Pain 16:109-110
10. Aloisi AM, Ceccarelli I, Lupo C (1998) Behavioural and hormonal effects of restraint stress and formalin test in male and female rats. Brain Res Bull 47: 57-62
11. Fonnum F (1968) Choline acetyltransferase binding to and release from membranes. Biochem J 109:389-398
12. Luine VN, Renner KJ, Heady S, Jones KJ (1986) Age and sex-dependent decreases in ChAT in basal forebrain nuclei. Neurobiol Aging 7:193-198
13. Gibbs RB (1998) Impairment of basal forebrain cholinergic neurons associated with aging and long-term loss of ovarian function. Exp Neurol 151:289-302
14. Goudsmit E, Luine VN, Swaab DF (1990) Testosterone locally increases vasopressin content but fails to restore choline acetyltransferase activity in other regions in the senescent male rat brain. Neurosci Lett 112:290-296
15. Pan Y, Anthony M, Clarkson TB (1999) Effect of estradiol and soy phytoestrogens on choline acetyltransferase and nerve growth factor mRNAs in the frontal cortex and hippocampus of female rats. Proc Soc Exp Biol Med 221:118-125
16. Ceccarelli I, Casamenti F, Massafra C et al (1999) Effects of novelty and pain on behavior and hippocampal extracellular ACh levels in male and female rats. Brain Res 815:169-176
17. Moroni F, Malthe-Sorenssen D, Cheney DL, Costa E (1978) Modulation of ACh turnover in the septal-hippocampal pathway by electrical stimulation and lesioning. Brain Res 150:333-341
18. Vernadakis A, Kentroti S (1990) Opioids influence neurotransmitter phenotypic expression in chick embryonic neuronal cultures. J Neurosci Res 26:342-348

Chapter 7

Consciousness and Pain

C.R. Chapman, Y. Nakamura

Consciousness was once a topic that mainstream scientists would not address. In recent years, however, the study of consciousness has attracted a multidisciplinary following that includes neuroscientists, behavioral scientists, evolutionary biologists, computer scientists, mathematicians, physicists, and philosophers [1-3]. Consciousness researchers pursue the question of how the physical brain can produce phenomenal reality, how the brain organizes a coherent awareness from the chaos of sensory input, the sense of self, the mechanisms of blind sight and blind touch, and myriad other phenomena of awareness. Among the questions that consciousness researchers must ask are "What is the nature of pain? Why do we have the ability of feel pain? Why does pain hurt?"

Pain research can bring many puzzling phenomena to the multidisciplinary consciousness research arena. Most pain depends upon and results from nociception – the nonconscious neural traffic that signals tissue trauma within the nervous system. However, nociception and pain are not equivalents. Some nociceptive signaling does not reach consciousness but rather provokes motor or sympathetic nervous system reflexes at the level of the spinal cord. Moreover, some chronic pain states do not involve nociception, e.g., phantom limb pain and central pain states (pains originating in damage to the central nervous system [4].

More fundamentally, there is a poor fit between tissue trauma and pain. In the area of acute pain, given a similar magnitude of tissue trauma (e.g., surgery), different persons report a wide range of pain magnitudes, respond differently to treatment, and display different levels of functional impairment in response to unrelieved pain [5-7]. There is a wide range of analgesic requirements for patients following surgery.

Poor fit also characterizes the relationship of tissue trauma and chronic pain, a complex condition with a debilitating awareness of bodily injury that may persist beyond the normal healing of tissue damage. Tissue pathology may be the source of chronic back pain for some patients, but similar pathology exists in other people without causing any pain. A magnetic resonance imaging (MRI) scan study [8] documented that about 35% of people without pain clearly have significant spine pathology. Conversely, chronic pain can, and often does, exist in the absence of detectable physical pathology [9]. It has become clear that the study of nociception is necessary, but not sufficient, for an understanding of pain.

For these reasons, there is mutual benefit in the collaboration of pain researchers and consciousness investigators. Pain research may be able to accelerate progress toward its ultimate goal of creating a comprehensive and coherent knowledge base on pain by strategically fitting an overarching consciousness research framework to its multidisciplinary efforts. This paper (a) provides a definition of consciousness suitable for pain researchers, (b) considers emerging research on functional brain imaging during pain, and (c) suggests a consciousness research framework for pain that may help accelerate progress in the pain field.

What is Consciousness?

Because consciousness research is multidisciplinary and multifocal, many definitions of consciousness exist. Most investigators agree that consciousness is an emergent feature of the brain, a dynamical, self-organizing process operating in a distributed neural network. As a product of evolution, consciousness increases the repertoire of behaviors and the functional capability of the individual. Viewed neurologically, consciousness has certain on-off features (coma, sleep, anesthesia), but it is more useful to think of it as graded, varying in degree of activation or arousal. This gradation is like the degree of illumination of a theatrical stage, upon which various characters appear. This stage analogy is a part of the theater metaphor in Baars' global workspace model of consciousness [10]. From moment to moment, specific mental objects emerge into the spotlight of consciousness and then fade into the background. Consciousness entails a constant ebb and flow in focus.

Many important brain functions are preconscious or nonconscious. That is, they occur outside of focal awareness, require faster computation than conscious thought can muster, are nonlinear, and often are nonverbal. Prototypical examples include the use of over-learned skills such as riding a bicycle or using the rules of linguistic grammar. We accomplish our most important work and insights below the level of consciousness, delivering the final product as an insight. What we call intuition and creativity result from nonconscious processing.

No existing definition of consciousness fits the needs of investigators in diverse scientific fields and philosophers of varied persuasions. For immediate purposes, we offer the following definition as a basis for fitting pain research into the framework of consciousness studies: consciousness is an emergent, self-organizing feature of brain activity that makes possible complex, adaptive interactions with the internal and external environments and self-reference in those environments.

What is Pain?

The standard definition of pain derives from the work of the International Association for the Study of Pain (IASP). According to the IASP, "Pain [is] an unpleasant sensory and emotional experience associated with actual or potential tissue damage, or described in terms of such damage" ([11], p. 250]. This definition emphasizes the role of affect as an intrinsic component of pain. Nonetheless, a sensory neurophysiological framework has dominated pain research from its inception and shaped the understanding of philosophers and the lay public. The strictest neurophysiological concept of pain holds that it is a sensory message of peripheral tissue trauma, specifically and accurately coded in peripheral nerves, transmitted in specific central pathways, and decoded in the brain. Hudson [12] recently offered an elegant model that expands and extends classical thinking in this framework to include prefrontal cortex. Who or what interprets the signals that complete their journey from periphery to cortex is never formally specified in papers on the brain and pain, but an implicit Cartesian dualism pervades the literature. The basic neurophysiological model tacitly assumes that a conscious entity somehow receives and interprets tissue trauma alarm signals.

Contemporary understanding of pain in medical practice also reflects a Cartesian perspective: the brain detects and perceives pathological bodily processes passively and somewhat mechanically. This perspective has deep historical roots. Viewing the body and mind as separate entities, early philosophers and scientists held that pain is a specific modality – a straight-through sensory projection system that moves injury signals from damaged tissue to the brain where the mind grasps them. This perspective went unchallenged for two centuries, and it still exerts considerable influence today. Scientists and physicians alike assumed, until the 1960s, that tissue trauma activates specific receptors and that signals of tissue trauma follow specific pain pathways through the spinal cord to a pain center in the brain [13]. Today, converging information from classical neurophysiology and functional brain imaging is opening a new understanding.

Pain and Functional Brain Imaging

Before functional brain imaging research came on the scene, neurophysiologists felt secure in their understanding of pain, and others, such as clinicians and behavioral scientists, assumed that classical neurophysiology was the only window of pain mechanisms. Nociceptive signals made their way to the dorsal horn of the spinal cord, moved on to the thalamus, and reached the somatosensory cortex, where they entered the mind through a still unspecified process. In less than a decade, functional brain imaging research, particularly positron emission tomography (PET) investigation of brain metabolic activity and functional magnetic resonance imaging (fMRI) investigation of brain metabolic activity, has revealed massive distributed processing in brain areas including, but not limited to, somatosensory pathways. Some of the active areas are in the limbic brain, which implicates emotion in pain perception. Moreover, converging evidence from neurophysiology is also showing that, in addition to spinothalamocortical pathways, brainstem and limbic structures are involved in pain [14].

The complexity of the central processing of painful events is striking. In people experiencing pain, distributed processing involves the hypothalamus, internal capsule (lenticular nucleus), the anterior cingulate, the insular cortex, the thalamus, the somatosensory cortices, the superior and inferior frontal cortex, the straight gyrus, and the cerebellar vermis. For reviews of these findings see Hudson [12], Davis [15], Porro and Cavazutti [16], and Ingvar [17]. Functional brain imaging studies reveal that the limbic brain, the seat of emotion, undertakes a major part of the processing that builds the experience of pain. The emotional aspects of pain are invariably negative, and central noradrenergic pathways may play a role in building the disturbing emotional quality of pain [18].

Although the limited time resolution of some imaging technology prevents investigators from specifying which aspects of distributed processing are serial and which are parallel, these studies demonstrate unequivocally that extensive distributed processing occurs in multiple areas of the brain. At present, investigators are struggling to assign pain-related patterns of activation to specific brain functions and to extend such mappings to an explanation of how we hurt [19]. The functional brain imaging observations do not relate readily to the knowledge base that neurophysiologists have built by studying nociceptive transduction, transmission and modulation. Conventional information flow concepts handily explain the generation and transmission of signals of tissue trauma in the periphery and spinal cord, but they provide insufficient explanations for the complexity of higher-order central nervous system activity during pain. A careful sensory neurophysiological investigation that strays from the spinothalamic pathway quickly becomes lost in a huge and complex maze of reciprocal connections. The processes that play out across the central nervous system structures still elude understanding.

Emerging data from studies involving functional brain imaging of pain suggest that nociceptive messages do not pass unnoticed on their way to sensory realization. Instead, they generate a cascade of other messages that engender complex patterns of processing throughout the brain, some of which may entail feedback-dependent neuroendocrine messaging [20]. Moreover, some, but probably not all, of these processes feed forward to shape the emotional and cognitive as well as sensory aspects of the pain experience. Patterns of brain response may well depend not only on sensory modality but also on the context of ongoing brain activity. If brain activation is context dependent, the goal of mapping brain activity related to pain may prove more difficult and complicated than we currently imagine.

It is becoming increasingly clear that pain researchers lack a framework for drawing a strong inference from functional brain imaging observations of pain. Strong theory could expedite and guide this line of inquiry. We propose that consciousness research can contribute such a framework.

Approaching Pain from a Consciousness Perspective

Much consciousness research makes use of the concepts of decentralized, dynamical, nonlinear self-organization processes and complexity [21]. Biology offers thousands of examples of how organisms, ranging from colonies of bacteria to flocks of birds, organize themselves as leaderless collectives in the course of adapting to their environments. Crowd behavior, traffic jams, and culture itself are human aspects of the self-organization process. Nonlinear systems dynamics, as a field, lends itself as a descriptive framework for self-organizing processes [22, 23]. It views seemingly chaotic phenomena as complex systems.

The concept of emergence is another building block for many workers in the consciousness field [24, 25]. Emergence simply means that combining certain elements produces a complex system that possesses properties lacking in the individual elements and unpredictable from knowledge of the individual elements. Expressed as a familiar cliché, the whole is different from the sum of the parts. Atoms of hydrogen and atoms of oxygen at room temperature are gases, but when combined, the property of liquidity emerges. Emergent properties are just this – the spontaneous emergence of hitherto nonexistent features. The apparent intelligence of an ant hill is an emergent property of the collective. No individual ant is intelligent, and nothing we know about individual ants allows us to predict the astonishing intelligence that the colony displays. The concept of emergent property offers a way out of the constrained thinking of Cartesian clockwork mechanics.

Inherent in the concept of emergence is the importance of hierarchy in scientific endeavor [26]. Interesting, unprecedented properties emerge as one goes from lower to higher levels of scientific inquiry. Emergent properties often define domains of study by specifying the boundaries of a given paradigm. The neurophysiologist who attempts to explain subjective reality from the activity of neurons and circuits in the brain simply comes to the edge of the neurophysiologist's territory. To work with subjective reality, one needs the paradigms of psychology.

Curiously, researchers engaged at one level of scientific inquiry tend to ignore the efforts of colleagues working at higher or lower levels and sometimes consider them misguided or busy wasting time and effort. The ultimate goal of reductionistic science, of course, is to build knowledge bases at each level and then achieve explanatory bridges across levels. Consciousness research recognizes the importance of building knowledge and bridges at all levels.

Many of the phenomena that pain researchers study are self-organizing, complex systems – sleeping nociceptors, dorsal horn modulation, and opioid tolerance are but a few. Such systems change in response to changing information. They vary in complexity, and simpler systems can nest within systems that are more complex. One measure of complexity is a system's requirements for multiple levels of description; the more ways one can look at a system, then the more complex it is.

One of the intriguing properties of self-organizing systems is their ability to sustain their basic patterns despite changes in information. Several models of self-organization address this feature. *Autopoiesis* refers to self-reproduction and maintenance of form with time and change. Varela, Maturana and Uribe [27] introduced an autopoietic model to describe systems that (a) maintain their defining organization over time despite environmental perturbation and structural change and (b) regenerate their components in the course of their operation. All living systems, by their standard, qualify as autopoietic systems. Importantly, every system has as one of its features an observer (not necessarily a conscious observer) that distinguishes between itself and others and between itself and objects in the environment (e.g., the immune system appears to have a nonconscious observer).

Another important property of self-organizing systems is that they relate in one way or another to other systems. The realm in which a system exists (its environment) is its *domain*. Dynamical systems constantly engage in self-regulation and self-reference within the constraints of their domains. Human brains are complex, dynamical systems that exist in relationships of continuous adaptation to the bodies they inhabit, the external environment, and other brains [22]. They exhibit autopoiesis and have as a feature an observer (a sense of self). Damasio's three levels of the sense of self (proto-self, core self and autobiographical self) suggest a complex, heirarchally organized observer within the brain [28].

Self-organization and emergence are two sides of the same coin. Self-organizing processes lead to emergence. Emergent phenomena are typically self-organizing. We suggest that some pain states are emergent phenomena that result from changes in self-organizational processes.

Towards a Unified Framework for Understanding Consciousness and Pain

As the functional brain imaging studies cited above show, the brain displays multifocal, parallel and complex central processing during the experience of pain. Therefore, we propose that dynamically distributed processing in large-scale networks, operating in parallel, integrates and synthesizes noxious signaling and other products of central processing to construct the contents of consciousness. Pain is but one aspect of this complex, constantly self-organizing process, and yet it is a prominent aspect because of its strong aversive quality.

How parallel, distributed processing in various brain regions constructs the awareness of pain and the associated suffering is still uncertain. We suggest that parallel distributed processing initiated by tissue trauma involves self-organized response patterns and that dynamically emerging response patterns, rather than pathways, are the proper focus for interpreting functional brain imaging observations of people experiencing pain.

The following processes seem to characterize central processing associated with pain: (1) multiple central response patterns compete for dominance (this is an evolutionary theory concept of cell assemblies, well-articulated by Calvin [29]; see Taylor [30] for similar ideas about neural networks); (2) sensory signaling integrates with expectation and other components of memory networks, various associations and motives appropriate to the immediate situation, and the long range goals of the person; and (3) self-organization forms a coherent whole from the sum of the many parts of the distributed processing. This coherent whole is dynamical by nature: the contents of consciousness evolve constantly, but (apart from dreaming) they maintain coherence.

The human brain, unless unconscious, constantly creates ordered perception from multi-modal sensory chaos. Sensory signals from the external world occur together with sensory signals from the somatic environment, and these combine with memory and multiple associations before awareness emerges. Most of the information potentially available in the brain does not enter consciousness because the brain selectively filters the sensory barrage, selecting certain information sources and rejecting others. Top down influences such as expectation, motivation, and selective attention guide this process, which constructs coherent patterns of experience. Pain, viewed in this context, is inherently complex and multi-dimensional. It is the product of a complex system, open to modeling in terms of nonlinear systems dynamics.

We have advocated adopting a nonlinear systems dynamical framework for the study of pain as a phenomenon of consciousness [20]. Our model, nested within this broader framework, contends that the brain constructs the experience of pain. The challenges of explaining why we sometimes fail to experience pain despite tissue trauma, why some people suffer greatly from pain that has no apparent origin, and why the brain sometimes produces pain when it is damaged are formidable. It seems clear that the current paradigm for the study of nociception will not answer these and other pressing questions. Although the application of nonlinear systems dynamics to the study of pain involve many uncertainties and will require a pioneer spirit, the scientific and humanitarian payoffs for progress in this endeavor are great.

References

1. Dennett D (1991) Consciousness explained. Little Brown, Boston
2. Greenfield SA (1995) Journey to the centers of the mind: toward a science of consciousness. WH Freeman, New York
3. Hameroff SR, Kaszniak AW, Scott AC (1996) Toward a science of consciousness. MIT Press, Cambridge
4. Chapman CR, Stillman M (1996) Pathological pain. In: Kruger L (ed) Pain and touch, 2nd edn. Academic, New York, pp 315-342
5. Jacobsen PB, Butler RW (1996) Relation of cognitive coping and catastrophizing to acute pain and analgesic use following breast cancer surgery. J Behav Med 19:17-29
6. Schechter NL, Bernstein BA, Beck A et al (1991) Individual differences in children's response to pain: role of temperament and parental characteristics. Pediatrics 87:171-177
7. Chapman CR, Hill HF, Saeger L, Gavrin J (1990) Profiles of opioid analgesia in humans after intravenous bolus administration: alfentanil, fentanyl and morphine compared on experimental pain. Pain 43:47-55
8. Jensen MC, Brant-Zawadzki MN, Obuchowski N et al (1994) Magnetic resonance imaging of the lumbar spine in people without back pain [see comments]. N Engl J Med 331:69-73
9. Turk DC (1996) Biopsychosocial perspective on chronic pain. In: Gatchel RJ, Turk DC (eds) Psychological approaches to pain management: a practitioner's handbook. Guilford Press, New York, pp 3-32
10. Baars BJ (1997) In the theater of consciousness. Oxford University Press, New York
11. Merskey H (1979) Pain terms: a list with definitions and a note on usage. Recommended by the International Association for the Study of Pain (IASP) Subcommittee on Taxonomy. Pain 6:249-252
12. Hudson AJ (2000) Pain perception and response: central nervous system mechanisms. Can J Neurol Sci 27:2-16
13. Bonica JJ (1953) The management of pain. Lea and Febiger, Philadelphia
14. Willis WD, Westlund KN (1997) Neuroanatomy of the pain system and of the pathways that modulate pain. J Clin Neurophysiol 14:2-31
15. Davis KD (2000) The neural circuitry of pain as explored with functional MRI. Neurol Res 22:313-317
16. Porro CA, Cavazzuti M (1996) Functional imaging studies of the pain system in man and animals. Prog Brain Res 110:47-62

17. Ingvar M (1999) Pain and functional imaging. Philos Trans R Soc Lond B Biol Sci 354:1347-1358
18. Chapman CR (1996) Limbic processes and the affective dimension of pain. In: Carli G, Zimmerman M (eds) Towards the neurobiology of chronic pain, vol 110. Elsevier, New York, pp 63-81
19. Casey KL (1996) Match and mismatch: identifying the neuronal determinants of pain. Ann Intern Med 124:995-998
20. Chapman CR, Nakamura Y (1999) A passion of the soul: an introduction to pain for consciousness researchers. Conscious Cogn 8:391-422
21. Resnick M (1995) Beyond the centralized mindset. J Learning Sci 5:1-22
22. Freeman WJ (1995) Societies of brains. Lawrence Erlbaum Associates, Hillsdale, NJ
23. Bar-Yam Y (1997) Dynamics of complex systems. Addison-Wesley, Reading, MA
24. Baas NA (1996) A framework for higher order cognition and consciousness. In: Hameroff SR, Kaszniak AW, Scott AC (eds) Toward a science of consciousness. MIT Press, Cambridge, pp 633-648
25. Scott AC (1996) The hierarchical emergence of consciousness. In: Hameroff SR, Kaszniak AW, Scott AC (eds) Toward a science of consciousness. MIT Press, Cambridge, pp 659-671
26. Scott AC (1995) Stairway to the mind. Springer, New York
27. Varela FG, Maturana HR, Uribe R (1974) Autopoiesis: the organization of living systems, its characterization and a model. Curr Mod Biol 5:187-196
28. Damasio AR (1999) The feeling of what happens: body and emotions in the making of consciousness. Harcourt Brace, New York
29. Calvin WH (1987) The brain as a Darwin machine. Nature 330:33-34
30. Taylor JG (1996) A competition for consciousness. Neurocomputing 11:271-296

Chapter 8

Visceral Pain Mechanisms

M.A. GIAMBERARDINO, J. VECCHIET, G. AFFAITATI, L. VECCHIET

Introduction

Pain from the internal organs has traditionally been investigated less than somatic pain, mostly due to the more difficult access to visceral than to superficial body structures [1]. As a consequence, mechanisms of this form of pain were scarcely known for a long time. In recent years, however, due to the exponential increase in sophisticated technological devices and procedures for testing sensory function both in humans and animals, significant advances in the understanding of the pathophysiology of pain from internal organs have been made [2].

The first part of this chapter provides a description of the modalities of noxious stimulation and structures involved in the transmission of nociceptive signals in the viscera and illustrates the main characteristics of visceral pain in the clinical setting. The second part deals with the interpretation of the most important phenomena related to the symptom, as based on the most recent research findings in the field. At the end of the chapter, a special section is devoted to the controversial issue of gender differences in visceral pain.

Visceral Nociception: Peripheral and Central Pathways

Adequate Stimuli

Viscera have long been considered insensitive to pain as they do not normally respond to most of the stimuli that are algogenic for somatic structures, such as cutting, pinching or burning [3]. Stimuli adequate enough to induce pain at the visceral level are, instead: abnormal distension and contraction of the muscle walls of hollow viscera, abrupt stretching of capsules of solid organs (such as the liver or the spleen), abrupt anoxemia of smooth muscles, traction or compression of ligaments and vessels, formation and accumulation of pain-producing substances, direct action of chemical substances (particularly important for organs such as the stomach or oesophagus), necrosis of some structures (such as myocardium or pancreas), and inflammatory states.

Contraction of a hollow viscus under isometric conditions (as occurs when the outlet of the viscus is obstructed) produces pain of much greater severity than that produced by contraction in isotonic conditions. This is, in fact, the mechanism of colic (renal/ureteral, biliary, etc.), which is amongst the most intense forms of pain.

Inflammatory states cause visceral pain directly as well as indirectly by sensitizing visceral tissues to non-painful stimuli. Algogenic substances such as kinins, 5-hydroxytryptamine, histamine, prostaglandins, and potassium released locally in the inflamed area of visceral tissues are probable mediators of the painful signals from inflamed viscera [4].

The extent of internal damage produced by various stimuli at the visceral level has no direct relationship to the occurrence and intensity of visceral pain [5]. Typical examples of this assumption are silent myocardial infarction, on the one hand – in which extensive damage to the cardiac muscle occurs without any pain perceived by the patient – and angina, on the other – in which pain occurs in the presence of ischaemia but in the absence of any damage to the myocardium.

Visceral sensitivity to pain also depends on the type of internal organ involved. Solid viscera are the least sensitive, followed, in order, by the wall of hollow organs and the serosal membranes, which are the most sensitive of all [6].

Visceral Nociceptors

The characteristics of visceral receptors involved in signalling painful events have long been a matter of scientific debate [7]. According to some researchers, painful stimuli in internal organs are encoded in the discharge of receptors with no background activity that respond only to high-intensity stimulation, i.e. specific nociceptors or "high threshold receptors", which are similar to those described in the skin, muscle, and joints ("specificity theory"). Other authors claim that noxious events in viscera are encoded in the intensity of discharge of the same population of receptors which also respond to innocuous events ("intensity theory") (see [6, 7]. Experimental evidence indeed exists for a specific role being played by both kinds of mechanisms in the viscera. "High threshold receptors" sensitive to mechanical stimuli have been identified in many visceral domains, i.e. ureter, biliary system, small instestine, uterus, veins, lungs and airways, while "intensity receptors" that encode for noxious stimuli have been documented in the testes. Organs such as the heart, oesophagus, colon and urinary bladder harbour both kinds of receptors [2, 6, 7]. The controversy between intensity and specificity theories applied to the visceral domain has thus subsided in recent years, since it has now become apparent that the two mechanisms of receptor activation are not mutually exclusive. The relative importance of the two possibly varies according to the individual visceral district involved [8].

A third category of receptors which play an important role in visceral nociception is that of the so-called "silent (or sleeping) nociceptors". These receptors are either unresponsive or have a very high activation threshold. However, they can be "awakened", i.e. sensitized by prolonged noxious stimulation, leading to inflammation or frank damage in tissues. Receptors with these characteristics were originally identified in joints [9] as units that could only be activated after the induction of experimental arthritis. They were subsequently also identified in viscera, i.e. the urinary bladder, and recently have also been recorded in the heart [2, 7]. Under conditions of experimental inflammation from chemical irritants in the urinary bladder, in fact, many unmyelinated and initially unresponsive afferents were sensitized, generating ongoing activity and, in some cases, also showing a novel mechanosensitivity (i.e. recruitment of mechanically insensitive afferents) [10].

Visceral Afferent Fibres

Sensory fibres in the viscera are constituents of the spinal and cranial nerves, having their cell bodies in the posterior root ganglia of spinal nerves or the ganglia of cranial nerves. Their distal processes mostly have the same course as sympathetic and also parasympathetic nerves, reaching the viscera while their central processes pass via the dorsal (and occasionally the ventral) roots. Although the size and range of these fibres are comparable to that of cutaneous fibres, there is a considerably higher proportion of small fibres, with A-delta being predominat among the A fibres. Furthermore, the ratio between A and C fibres, which is approximately 1:2 in the dorsal root, is only 1:8 (or 1:10) in visceral nerves [4].

The density of innervation of the viscera by spinal afferents is small compared with the density of afferent innervation in the skin and probably also in many deep somatic structures. Visceral afferents represent 5%-15% of the neuronal cell bodies in the dorsal root ganglia at the spinal segments receiving maximal visceral afferent input. The relative number of spinal neurons that respond to visceral afferent input at these same spinal segments, however, ranges from 56% to 75%. Therefore, a few visceral afferent fibres can activate many neurons in the spinal cord through extensive functional divergence [5,6].

Central Projection of Visceral Afferent Fibres

The second-order neurons that receive visceral inputs are mostly located in laminae I and V of the dorsal horn as well as in the ventral horn of the spinal cord, and they are also activated by somatic inputs. Viscerosomatic convergence is, thus, the rule in the central nervous system. According to Cervero [11], the viscerosomatic neurons in the spinal cord can be subdivided into two categories: (a) a minority of neurons mainly situated in the superficial dorsal horn, with a limited, ipsilateral visceral input plus a cutaneous input (with restricted receptive fields activated only by noxious stimuli) and subjected to descending inhibitory control. They project to the brain via spinothalamic pathways; and (b) a majority of neurons situated in the deep dorsal and ventral horn, with a diffuse and bilateral visceral input and a somatic input, often from deep tissues (with large and multireceptive fields), and subjected to descending excitatory and inhibitory control. The excitatory control probably originates from the rostral medullary centres. A number of these neurons project to the reticular formation of the brainstem.

In addition to viscero-somatic convergence in the spinal cord, viscero-visceral convergence also exists onto the same second-order neurons. Convergence has, for instance, been documented between colon/rectum, bladder, vagina and uterine cervix (as well as from the skin) and between gallbladder and heart in electrophysiological studies in animals [12,13].

Both viscero-somatic and viscero-visceral convergence are maintained at the supraspinal level (e.g. brainstem, thalamus, and cerebral cortex) [6].

Visceral Pain Phenomena in the Clinical Setting

Visceral pain is encountered very frequently in clinical practice; it represents, in fact, a major reason for seeking medical care. It manifests with different characteristics, depending on the stage of the underlying disease, i.e. it tends to follow a temporal evolution [2]. In the first phases of an algogenic process from an internal organ, the pain is vague and poorly localized, always perceived in the same site whatever the viscus in question, i.e. the midline of thorax or abdomen, anteriorly or posteriorly, mostly the lowest sternal or epigastric regions. The quality of the sensation is dull, often not even reported as pain, but just as a sense of malaise, discomfort, or constriction in the described region. Marked neurovegetative signs constantly accompany the symptom: nausea, vomiting, pallor, sweating, alvus disturbances, changes in heart rate and blood pressure, etc. Emotional reactions are often present, such as anguish, anxiety and a sense of impending death. The intensity of the symptom in this phase (phase of *true visceral pain*) varies from slight to unbearable and is not modified by additional stimuli applied to the painful area. The duration is always limited, i.e. from minutes to a few hours, after which the pain either ceases or changes its characteristics, that is, it becomes referred to somatic structures of the body which vary, depending on the viscus involved. In the phase of referred pain, in fact, the symptom is normally perceived in areas neuromerically connected with the viscus in question; it is sharper and better defined, no longer accompanied by emotional reactions and marked neurovegetative signs. In this phase, the pain may or may not be associated with a condition of secondary hyperalgesia (increased sensitivity to painful stimuli) of the tissues in the painful area, so that two types of referred pain from viscera can be distinguished: *referred pain without hyperalgesia* and *referred pain with hyperalgesia*. Referred pain without hyperalgesia is also called irradiated segmental pain. Additional stimuli exerted on the area of referral do not increase the symptom and the pain threshold is not decreased. Infiltration of local anaesthetic in the painful area produces no effect.

Referred pain with hyperalgesia is also called true parietal pain. Additional stimuli applied onto the painful area increase the painful sensation and the pain threshold is normally decreased. The hyperalgesia most frequently involves the muscle layer, but often extends upwards to also involve the subcutaneous tissue and the skin, in the case of repeated and/or longlasting algogenic processes [6].

Muscle hyperalgesia has been documented in the areas of referred pain from the viscera in terms of a significant decrease in pain thresholds to both mechanical and electrical muscle stimuli in a number of clinical studies on patients affected with different visceral pathologies (e.g. renal colics, biliary colics, and primary dysmenorrhoea) [14-19]. This hyperalgesia appeared to be an early process, as it tended to manifest as early as the first visceral episodes, was accentuated in extent by the repetition of the visceral pains and lasted for a long time, i.e. it not only outlasted the spontaneous pain from the internal organ, but sometimes also the presence itself of the primary focus in the viscus. In patients affected with urinary calculosis it was in fact often detectable even a long time after the stone had been expelled. In addition to the sensory changes (hyperalgesia), the somatic tissues in the areas of referred pain from viscera are also often the site of trophic changes, mostly in terms of increased thickness and consistency of the subcutaneous tissue and decreased thickness and section area of muscles (tendency to muscle atrophy) [3]. These phenomena were documented via clinical procedures but also precisely quantified through ultrasound evaluation in patients [19, 20].

In algogenic conditions affecting internal organs, hyperalgesic phenomena are very frequent, not only involving the somatic areas of referral, as just described, but also affecting the visceral structures themselves [1, 2]. A given internal organ can, in fact, become hyperalgesic due to local inflammation and/or excess (repetitive-prolonged) stimulation (*visceral hyperalgesia*). This is a form of primary hyperalgesia, i.e. involving the site of injury. In the clinical setting, hypersensitivity due to inflammation indeed appears to be one of the most common and best known forms of visceral hyperalgesia. Typical examples are represented by pain upon ingestion of food or liquids at the level of the oesophagus or stomach when the mucosa is inflamed or by pain upon bladder distension from inflammatory processes of the lower urinary tract, for instance those accompanying common infections such as cystitis.

Phenomena of visceral hyperalgesia can also occur as a result of an algogenic interaction between different visceral domains. This is the case of hyperalgesia of one visceral organ which becomes clinically manifest because of an algogenic condition of another viscus whose segmental afferent innervation is partially overlapping (*viscero-visceral hyperalgesia*). It is not unusual to observe in the clinic that patients with ischaemic heart disease who are also affected with gallbladder calculosis complain of a higher number of anginal attacks than patients with ischaemic heart disease and a normal gallbladder [gallbladder and heart have a partially overlapping central projection (at T5 level)]. Another example is the interaction between pathologies of the urinary tract and female reproductive organs, such as urinary calculosis and dysmenorrhoea (for female reproductive organs and urinary tract, common segments: T10-L1). Women with dysmenorrhoea experience more painful urinary colic episodes from calculosis than non-dysmenorrhoeic women in a comparable period of time, and during the menstrual cycle the temporal patterns of the episodes differ between the two groups. Specifically, dysmenorrhoeic women are significantly more likely to have a colic during their perimenstrual phase and at ovulation than are women without severe dysmenorrhoea [1, 2]. These observations suggest that colic pain from the urinary tract in fertile women is preferentially manifested in periods of the cycle when the input from the female reproductive organs is enhanced because of pelvic congestion (around either menstruation or ovulation).

In addition to a higher number of urinary colics, dysmenorrhoeic women with respect to normal women also present a much greater degree of referred muscle hyperalgesia at the lumbar level, i.e. in the area of pain referral from the urinary tract, than non-dysmenorrhoeic women who have experienced a comparable number of colics. Thus, referred hyperalgesia from the urinary tract is also notably enhanced by the concomitant presence of the inflammatory condition of the reproductive organs.

Mechanisms of Visceral Pain Phenomena

True visceral pain is usually felt around the midline because visceral organs are supplied with afferents bilaterally; exceptions are the caecum, ascending colon, descending and sigmoid colon, kidneys, and ureters, whose innervation is unilateral or predominantly so [4]. The poor localization and diffuse nature of the pain result from the low density of sensory innervation of the viscera, together with the extensive functional divergence of the visceral input within the central nervous system. A contribution to the relative aspecificity of the visceral sensation in this phase (i.e. the difficulty in identifying its source) is also made by the viscero-visceral convergence at the central level.

Referred pain without hyperalgesia is normally interpreted on the basis of the convergence-projection theory, based on extensive experimental evidence of the convergence at the central level (spinal and supraspinal centres) of visceral and somatic afferent fibres onto the same neurons. The message from the viscera would thus be interpreted by higher brain centres as coming from the somatic structure because of mnemonic traces of previous experiences of somatic pain [3,5].

Referred pain with hyperalgesia, by far more common than the corresponding form without hyperalgesia, is more difficult to interpret and the simple convergence-projection theory does not appear adequate to account for it. There is at present an increasing body of evidence, in experimental studies, for the contribution of central mechanisms to the generation of the hyperalgesia [2]. The massive afferent barrage from the visceral domain would trigger a number of neuroplastic changes in the CNS, involving hyperactivity and hyperexcitability of sensory neurons (convergent viscero-somatic), so that the normal input from the somatic periphery of pain referral would have an enhanced effect at the central level (convergence-facilitation).

This phenomenon of central sensitization involving viscero-somatic convergent neurons has indeed been documented in cases of referred hyperalgesia from viscera in electrophysiological studies in animal models of the condition [21]. One such model was originally set up by our group and subsequently employed by other laboratories [22, 23]. It is a model of experimental ureteric calculosis in rats, which mimics the condition of urinary colics and referred lumbar muscle hyperalgesia in humans. Rats in which an artificial stone is formed in the upper third of one ureter show behavioural signs indicative of both direct visceral pain (multiple complex "ureteral crises" over 4 days postoperatively) and referred hyperalgesia of the ipsilateral oblique musculature (decrease in vocalization thresholds to electrical muscle stimulation for over a week postoperatively). As in patients, the extent of the referred muscle hyperalgesia is correlated with the number of painful visceral episodes and outlasts the signs of spontaneous pain, sometimes even beyond the presence of the stone in the urinary tract. In fact, this hypersensitivity is often detectable up to the last day of evaluation even in rats which proved to have eliminated the stone through the urine, when examined autoptically. As already stated above, electrophysiological experiments at the spinal cord level in this animal model support the involvement of a central component in the production of referred hyperalgesia from viscera [24, 25]. Changes in the excitability and response properties of dorsal horn neurons which receive input from the hyperalgesic muscle in rats with artificial calculi have been found compared to control animals. A significantly increased percentage of dorsal horn neurons displayed a receptive field in the hyperalgesic muscle, a significantly higher percentage of which also showed ongoing activity. Neurons with muscle input also presented a decreased threshold of activation via mechanical stimuli. These changes were more marked in animals that had more visceral episodes and muscle hyperalgesia. Similar results were obtained by Roza et al. [23], employing this same model, in electrophysiological experiments in which they examined the characteristics of neurons processing information from the ureter (in calculosis rats versus rats with an intact ureter). These authors concluded that the presence of a ureteric stone evokes excitability changes of spinal neurons (enhanced background activity, greater number of ureter-driven cells, and decreased threshold of convergent somatic receptive fields) which likely account for the referred muscle hyperalgesia seen in rats with calculosis.

The fact that hyperalgesia often outlasts the presence of the "macroscopic" peripheral visceral focus in the clinical setting has led to the hypothesis that the central plastic changes, once established, may persist, becoming relatively independent of the primary triggering event [2]. However, the results of recent studies on ureter motility in rats with artificial ureteral calculosis (abnormal hypermotility persisting long after stone elimination) [22] suggest that a number of "clinically inapparent" peripheral visceral changes are likely to outlive the presence of the primary focus and thus maintain the state of central hyperexcitability via persistence of the peripheral drive.

The intervention of further mechanisms in the generation of referred hyperalgesia from viscera cannot be ruled out, i.e. the activation of a number of reflex arcs whose afferent branch is represented by the afferent fibres from the viscus and efferent branch by sympathetic and/or somatic efferences towards the tissues of the peripheral area of referral. These could be responsible for reflex sensitization of somatic nociceptors in this area, thus accounting for the hyperalgesia [3, 6]. The reflex arc hypothesis needs to be confirmed experimentally because, apart from some clinical evidence, not many other experimental studies have specifically addressed this issue. Some results in the rat model of ureteric calculosis would seem to indicate that a reflex mechanism could play a role in the generation of referred hyperalgesia from viscera. In fact, some degree of hyperactivity and hyperexcitability was found in neurons with input from the hyperalgesic muscle located in the intermediate region of the cord (level of the lowest thoracic segments), where the cells of origin of the sympathetic outflow are situated [24].

More studies are undoubtedly needed to test this hypothesis thoroughly. It seems plausible, though, especially in the light of the clinical evidence that the areas of referred pain from viscera are the site of trophic alterations in addition to the hyperalgesia; these objective changes cannot, in fact, be the result of purely central processes.

Visceral Hyperalgesia

Hyperalgesia from inflammation and/or excess stimulation is among the most extensively investigated phenomena of hypersensitivity from a visceral domain. To account for this form of hyperalgesia, mechanisms have been advocated which are similar to those involved in primary cutaneous hyperalgesia (at the site of an injury), i.e. mechanisms of both peripheral and central sensitization [2].

Peripheral sensitization involves a lowering in threshold of nociceptors. In internal organs, based on the present knowledge about the nature and characteristics of visceral sensory receptors, peripheral sensitization due to inflammation and/or repetitive-prolonged stimulation is likely to involve both a lowering in threshold of "high threshold receptors" and the bringing into play of previously unresponsive units ("silent nociceptors") [26].

The increased input to the CNS would then trigger neuroplastic changes which amplify the effects of every additional signal coming from the affected viscus. This process is known as central sensitization and involves phenomena of increased spontaneous activity of neurons, enlarged receptive field areas and an increase in response evoked by large and small-calibre primary afferent fibres [27].

The results of a number of experimental studies on animal models of visceral hyperalgesia point to a pivotal role played by *N*-metyl-*D*-aspartate (NMDA) receptors in mediating the state of central hyperexcitability. NMDA receptor agonists, in fact, have been shown to enhance visceral nociceptive responses and antagonists to prevent or inhibit these same responses due to experimental visceral inflammation in the rat produced via instillation of zymosan in the colon or of turpentine in the urinary bladder [28-30].

Viscero-Visceral Hyperalgesia

Viscero-visceral hyperalgesia is a complex form of hypersensitivity which is likely to be explained by more than one mechanism. Since this phenomenon takes place preferentially between visceral organs which share, at least in part, their central projection, it is plausible that phenomena of central sensitization play an important role. Hyperactivity and hyperexcitability could involve viscero-visceral convergent neurons at the central level. As already reported, in fact, viscero-visceral convergences have been documented in electrophysiological studies in animals, for instance between gallbladder and heart – which would explain the frequent interaction between pathologies of these two organs – and between colon/rectum, urinary bladder, vagina and uterine cervix – which would explain the clinical interaction between female reproductive organs and urinary tract. The increased input from one visceral domain could trigger changes in the excitability of these neurons and thus enhance the central effect of the input from the second visceral domain [2].

This hypothesis, however, needs to be verified experimentally, and other possible mechanisms might also be implicated. Accordingly, it would be of great importance to have available a reliable animal model of the condition of viscero-visceral interaction observed in patients. One such model has recently been set up which reproduces the characteristics of the viscero-visceral interaction between the female reproductive organs and the urinary tract. Our group combined the model of urinary calculosis in rats with a model of experimental endometriosis [12]. Endometriosis was chosen because it is a very frequent cause of secondary dysmenorrhoea in women [4]. Preliminary data in this model have shown that rats with experimental endometriosis plus urinary stones display a significantly higher number and duration of typical ureteral crises than rats with sham endometriosis plus urinary stones. In addition, they also show a much higher degree of referred muscle hyperalgesia than sham endometriosis rats. This appears to be the experimental counterpart of the clinical condition just described, and this model may be a useful tool for further investigation of underlying mechanisms.

Visceral Pain and Gender Issues

There is an increasing body of evidence, both in the clinical and experimental literature, for the existence of sex differences in the perception of pain [31], including visceral pain, although the direction of these differences is not always clear [32]. One first obvious difference between females and males regards their reproductive organs, which are, of course, sex-specific. Reproductive structures are mainly visceral organs; this means that women and men are subject to an array of different visceral algogenic pathologies in this area. Women are, however, much more prone than men to experience pain from their sex-specific organs, in part due to the higher complexity of their reproductive function. Women are thus subject to mild to severe recurrent forms of pain from the uterus (depending on whether they are dysmenorrhoeic) with the ovarian cycle during their fertile years, may undergo labour pain as well as several forms of visceral "after pains" following labour itself. They are also more prone than men to present visceral pain from the reproductive area because of frank pathologic events, such as ascending genital infections which, for anatomical reasons, can give rise more frequently in women than in men to states of persistent pain from the pelvic area.

If we consider internal organs common to the two sexes, here, again, women and men appear to differ. Firstly, there is a different prevalence of a number of painful algogenic conditions from viscera. Some of these conditions – mostly organic – predominantly affect men (e.g. coronary heart disease, at least before the age of 55 years), while others prevail in women (e.g. gallbladder pathologies). This is mainly because of different risk factors between the two sexes (e.g. for atherosclerosis or biliary calculosis) related to both hormonal status and lifestyle. Other conditions – mostly dysfunctional or without identifiable organic cause, such as irritable bowel syndrome or interstitial cystitis – appear to largely prevail in women because of a supposed higher susceptibility of the female sex to present the phenomenon of "visceral hyperalgesia", already described in a previous section. Even for the same visceral algogenic pathology, how symptoms present often differs between men and women, i.e. the clinical profile of the same pathologic entity can vary greatly in the two sexes. Visceral pain appears to be less predictive in women than in men of a specific visceral disease and would thus be more difficult to identify and treat. An example is coronary artery disease. Women seem to be more prone to silent ischaemia than men and, at the same time, also more prone to present with chest pain not motivated by coronary pathology.

Another difference between the two sexes regards the fact that women, but not men, are subject to fluctuations in the symptoms with the phases of the ovarian cycle during the fertile period of their life. The exact directions of these fluctuations are still a matter of debate, but a number of recent studies suggest an exacerbation of several pain conditions (especially those from internal organs) as the menstrual phase approaches.

Lastly, women seem to be more prone than men to present phenomena of viscero-visceral hyperalgesia between internal organs with partially overlapping innervation. An example is the already described interaction between the female reproductive organs and the urinary tract, two visceral domains that frequently are the site of potentially painful conditions throughout the course of a woman's life. These phenomena are likely to predispose women to more intricate and often more long-lasting painful experiences from internal organs as compared to men.

Conclusion

Mechanisms of visceral pain are more complex than those underlying pain from somatic structures. Some of them have been thoroughly clarified, while others – especially those related to the various forms of hyperalgesia linked to visceral nociception – are much less known and are currently under active investigation. In the patient affected with painful diseases of internal organs, several phenomena of visceral hypersensitivity can co-exist, which intermingle and give rise to intricate clinical pictures whose diagnosis and treatment are often difficult. Fully elucidating the mechanisms underlying these phenomena is thus of crucial importance for improving modalities of the approach to and management of the symptom in the clinical setting. It is hoped that further studies on experimental models which adequately reproduce the different clinical conditions will lead to a better understanding of visceral pain pathophysiology and, consequently, to the development of therapeutic strategies which are not merely aimed at treating symptoms.

References

1. Giamberardino MA (2000) Recent and forgotten aspects of visceral pain. Eur J Pain 3:77-92
2. Giamberardino MA (2000) Visceral hyperalgesia. In: Devor M, Rowbotham MC, Wiesenfeld-Halin Z (eds) Proceeding of the 9th World Congress on Pain, Progr Pain Res Ther. IASP Press, Seattle, pp 523-550
3. Procacci P, Zoppi M, Maresca M (1986) Clinical approach to visceral sensation. In: Cervero F, Morrison JFB (eds) Visceral sensation. (Progress in brain research, vol 67). Elsevier, Amsterdam, pp 21-28
4. Bonica JJ (ed) (1990) The Management of Pain. Lea and Febiger, Philadephia

5. Gebhart GF (ed) (1995) Visceral pain, (Progress in pain research and management, vol 5). IASP Press, Seattle
6. Giamberardino MA, Vecchiet L (1996) Pathophysiology of visceral pain. Curr Rev Pain 1:23-33
7. Cervero F (1996) Visceral nociceptors. In: Belmonte C, Cervero F (eds) Neurobiology of nociceptors. Oxford University Press, Oxford New York Tokyo, pp 220-240
8. Cervero F, Jänig W (1992) Visceral nociceptors: a new world order. Trends Neurosci 15:374-378
9. Schmidt RF, Schaible H-G, Messinger K et al (1994) Silent and active nociceptive structure, functions, and clinical implications. In: Gebhart GF, Hansmond DL, Jensen TS (eds) (Progress in pain research and management, vol. 0). IASP Press, Seattle, pp 213-250
10. Häbler H-J, Jänig W, Koltzenburg M (1990) Activation of unmyelinated afferent fibers by mechanical stimuli and inflammation of the urinary bladder in the cat. J Physiol 425:545-562
11. Cervero F (1994) Sensory innervation of the viscera: peripheral basis of visceral pain. Physiol Rev 74(1):95-138
12. Berkley KJ, Guilbaud G, Benoist JM, Gautron M (1993) Responses of neurons in and near the thalamic ventrobasal complex of the rat to stimulation of uterus, cervix, vagina, colon and skin. J Neurophysiol 69:557-568
13. Foreman RD (1999) Mechanisms of cardiac pain. Ann Rev Physiol 61:143-147
14. Vecchiet L, Giamberardino MA, Dragani L, Albe-Fessard D (1989) Pain from renal/ureteral calculosis: evaluation of sensory thresholds in the lumbar area. Pain 36:289-295
15. Vecchiet L, Giamberardino MA, Dragani L, Galletti R, Albe-Fessard D (1990) Referred muscular hyperalgesia from viscera: clinical approach. In: Lipton S, Tunks E, Zoppi M (ed) The pain clinic – Advances in pain research and therapy, vol 13. Raven Press, New York, pp 175-182
16. Vecchiet L, Giamberardino MA, de Bigontina P (1992) Referred pain from viscera: when the symptom persists despite the extinction of the visceral focus. In: Sicuteri F, Terenius L, Vecchiet L, Maggi CA (eds) Pain versus man (Advances in pain research and therapy, vol 20). Raven Press, New York, pp 101-110
17. Giamberardino MA, de Bigontina P, Martegiani C, Vecchiet L (1994) Effects of extracorporeal shock-wave lithotripsy on referred hyperalgesia from renal/ureteral calculosis. Pain 56:77-83
18. Giamberardino MA, Berkley KJ, Iezzi S et al (1997) Pain threshold variations in somatic wall tissues as a function of menstrual cycle, segmental site and tissue depth in non-dysmenorrheic women, dysmenorrheic women and men. Pain 71:187-197
19. Giamberardino MA, Affaitati G, Iezzi S, Vecchiet L (1999) Referred muscle pain and hyperalgesia from viscera. J Musculoskeletal Pain 7(1/2):61-69
20. Vecchiet L, Giamberardino MA (1998) Clinical and pathophysiological aspects of visceral hyperalgesia. In: De Vera JA, Parris W, Erdine S (eds) Management of pain. A world perspective III. Monduzzi, Bologna, pp 214-230
21. Giamberardino MA, Valente R, de Bigontina P, Vecchiet L (1995) Artificial ureteral calculosis in rats: behavioural characterization of visceral pain episodes and their relationship with referred lumbar muscle hyperalgesia. Pain 61:459-469
22. Laird JMA, Roza C, Cervero F (1997) Effects of artificial calculosis on rat ureter motility: peripheral contribution to the pain of ureteric colic. Am J Physiol 272:1409-1416
23. Roza C, Laird JMA, Cervero F (1998) Spinal mechanisms underlying persistent pain and referred hyperalgesia in rats with an experimental ureteric stone. J Neurophysiol 79:1603-1612

24. Giamberardino MA, Dalal A, Valente R, Vecchiet L (1996) Changes in activity of spinal cells with muscular input in rats with referred muscular hyperalgesia from ureteral calculosis. Neurosci Lett 203:89-92
25. Giamberardino MA, Valente R, Affaitati G, Vecchiet L (1997) Central neuronal changes in recurrent visceral pain. Int J Clin Pharmacol Res 17(2/3):63-66
26. Cervero F(1995) Visceral pain: mechanisms of peripheral and central sensitization. Ann Med 2: 235-239
27. Li J, Simone DA, Larson AA (1999) Windup leads to characteristics of central sensitization. Pain 79:75-82
28. Kolhekar R, Gebhart GF (1996) Modulation of spinal nociceptive transmission by NMDA receptor activation in the rat. J Neurophysiol 75:2344-2351
29. Coutinho SV, Meller ST, Gebhart GF (1996) Intracolonic zymosan produces visceral hyperalgesia in the rat that is mediated by spinal NMDA and non-NMDA receptors. Brain Res 736:7-15
30. Rice ASC, McMahon SB (1994) Pre-emptive intrathecal administration of an NMDA receptor antagonist (AP-5) prevents hyper-reflexia in a model of persistent visceral pain. Pain 57:335-340
31. Berkley KJ (1997) Sex differences in pain. Behav Brain Sci 20:371-380
32. Giamberardino MA (2000) Sex-related and hormonal modulation of visceral pain . In: Fillingim RB (ed) Sex, gender, and pain (Progress in pain research and management, Vol. 17). IASP Press, Seattle, pp 135-163

Chapter 9

PET-Scan and Electrophysiological Assessment of Neuromodulation Procedures for Pain Control

L. García-Larrea, R. Peyron, F. Mauguière, B. Laurent

The strong inhibitory influences that electrical stimulation of the nervous system can exert on pain transmission have been repeatedly demonstrated by experimental studies in animals [1-4], prompting the use of neurostimulation strategies for the relief of chronic pain in humans. As a logical corollary of the 'Gate control' theory [1, 5], which postulates that non-nociceptive signals tend to inhibit those conveyed by nociceptive pathways, the neural targets of stimulation procedures have been mostly the sensory pathways mediating transmission of non-noxious information, namely large afferent peripheral fibers, spinal dorsal columns and thalamic sensory nuclei (for both historical and up-to-date reviews see 6-9]. To a lesser extent brainstem structures exerting descending antinociceptive influences, such as the periaqueductal (PGA) and periventricular (PVG) grey matter have been also been used as targets [7]. Although stimulation of central motor fibers was also shown to inhibit afferent transmission in the dorsal horn [10, 11] and to produce analgesic effects in man [12] the use of motor cortex stimulation for pain control has been documented only recently [13]. Since then, the use of MCS for analgesic purposes is being increasingly used for refractory neuropathic pain [14-19].

Neurofunctional studies are useful in the clinical, pathophysiological and prognostic assessment of each of these procedures; however, the objectives of this type of evaluation differ in each of them: for example, spinal cord stimulation for chronic pain (SCS) is a well established and widely used procedure, the mechanisms of which are supported by a wealth of animal studies. Accordingly, neurophysiological studies in patients submitted to SCS are mainly devoted to demonstrating in man the existence of such mechanisms and to use the results as a guide for prognostic or follow up. Other neuromodulation procedures such as motor cortex stimulation are yielding encouraging clinical results, but the reasons accounting for their efficacy have not yet been elucidated. Clinical application in these cases remains therefore largely empirical, and neurofunctional assessment aims, first, to provide a neurobiological basis to explain their clinical effects, and second, to predict efficacy or optimise patient selection.

In this report we summarise our experience and that of others in the neurophysiological and neuroimaging assessment of spinal and brain neurostimulation. We concentrate on two types of intervention, both with analgesic purposes, namely (a) spinal and peripheral nerve stimulation and (b) motor cortex stimulation.

The Techniques for Evaluation

Nociceptive Spinal Reflexes

These are polysynaptic flexion responses subserving withdrawal from noxious stimuli. Described as early as 1910 by Sherrington [20], flexion nociceptive reflexes became a tool for human pain research after the observation that one of such responses (the "RIII" reflex) was consistently associated with a subjective sensation of pain [21] and that a high correlation existed between the threshold of this reflex and that of subjective pain [22, 23]. Similar correlations between segmental reflexes and ascending pain signals have been made in animals [24, 25] thus providing a conceptual basis for the utilisation of these responses in clinical practice.

In normal human, most consistent nociceptive reflexes are obtained in the hamstring muscles (notably biceps femoris), following stimulation of the ipsilateral sural nerve. However, pain-related reflexes can also be demonstrated in other lower limb muscles such as tibialis anterior and flexor hallucis longus, as well as in the upper limb (review in 26). Hugon [21] concluded that nociceptive responses after sural nerve stimulation were mediated by group III afferents (corresponding to A-delta fibers), which explains the label "RIII" commonly employed to refer to them.

Although of spinal origin, nociceptive reflexes are influenced by supraspinal activity. For example, drawing attention away from the noxious stimulus depresses both nociceptive reflexes and pain sensation [27, 28], suggesting that the analgesia obtained during attentional states includes a spinal mechanism. The analgesic properties of stress are also reflected in human spinal nociceptive responses, which increase their threshold under psychologically stressing conditions in a naloxone-reversible manner [29]. However, despite the extensive supraspinal influences on RIII, the spinal origin of this reflex is supported by its persistence after total spinal transection in man. It is nevertheless obvious that the simultaneous activation of long-loop reflexes contributing to RIII in normal humans cannot be ruled out, especially since lesions of the ascending nociceptive pathways are able to depress these responses [30].

Somatosensory Evoked Potentials

These are neuronal responses obtained in response to the stimulation of somatosensory receptors or somatic peripheral nerves. Somatosensory evoked potentials (SEPs) are usually obtained by applying electrical stimulation to the skin surface or nerves, thus bypassing peripheral receptors and activating the fibers directly (review in 31). SEPs to electrical stimulation explore in the periphery the activity of large myelinated fibers (A-Beta), and in the central nervous system that of dorsal column / medial lemniscus pathways which are not preferentially involved in pain transmission. More recently, SEPs to selective stimulation of thin myelinated (A-delta) and unmyelinated (C) fibers with laser beams have become available for clinical practice, thus allowing the assessment of responses vehiculated specifically by spinothalamic pain and temperature pathways (reviews in 32, 33). Both SEPs and laser-evoked potentials (LEPs) are useful for the diagnosis of pain pathophysiology, especially in neuropathic pain, and for the investigation of the mechanisms of neuromodulation used for pain relief. For the time being, while electrical SEPs allow the recording of peripheral, spinal and cortical responses, LEPs only permit the obtainment of cortical responses, but not of spinal or subcortical potentials. The cortical responses obtained with nociceptive stimulation reflect simultaneously the sensory and cognitive aspects of pain integration [34], and their interpretation may be more difficult than that of purely sensory responses such as subcortical SEPs.

Signal-processing techniques are needed to reveal stimulus-related somatosensory activity and eliminate background noise (i.e. voltage changes unrelated to the stimulus). Thus, individual responses to successive stimuli are averaged to improve the signal-to-noise ratio and enhance stimulus-related activity. The number of responses that need to be averaged to obtain good quality SEPs or LEPs varies as a function of both the size of the response and the amount of background noise, which in turn depends on both environmental noise and patient's relaxation. Typical figures are 30–100 consecutive stimuli for late cortical responses, 500–1500 for primary cortical potentials, and up to 2000 or more stimuli for subcortical (spinal or brainstem) SEPs.

Positron Emission Tomography (PET)

This technique of functional imaging measures concentrations of isotopes within a given body volume; such isotopes are carried by natural molecules which are usually injected and enter the brain via the blood stream. The *physical* variable that is directly measured by PET cameras is therefore the distribution of radioactivity, while the associated *physiological* variable depends on the molecule that carries the positron-emitting isotope. In studies of pain and pain modulation, where relatively rapid changes in activity are to be measured, isotopes with a short half-life are preferred, which allow repeated measurements in short amounts of time. One of the choice isotopes is 15O, with a half-life of about 2 minutes only, which can be included in natural molecules such as water or butanol and yields information on regional cerebral blood flow (rCBF). The so-called 'activation' PET studies investigate variations of rCBF specifically associated with a given task or a particular stimulus. Data interpretation is based on statistical comparisons of rCBF values obtained in two clinical or experimental situations, often labelled 'activated' and 'control' conditions. These are the measurements that will be dealt with in this lecture.

Measurement of rCBF has proven a sensitive, simple and versatile approach to functional brain mapping [35]. Local CBF increases reflect increases in local synaptic activity [36], and are equal to or greater than those observed in glucose metabolic rate. The short scan duration (50-90 seconds) and interscan interval (10-15 minutes) permit multiple studies in rapid succession. PET-scan studies have been mainly addressed to the study of brain responses to experimental pain in normals and clinical pain in patients (for a review see 37). In the context of neurostimulation procedures for pain, PET has been used by a number of teams to assess changes in rCBF associated with stimulation of the spinal cord [38], thalamic relay nuclei [39] and precentral cortex [40, 41].

Assessment of Neuromodulation Procedures for Pain

Spinal Cord Stimulation (SCS)

This technique has been used increasingly in the treatment of chronic neuropathic pain since its introduction in 1965. Important clinical requisites for successful SCS have been disclosed, such as that the stimulation-induced paresthesia must cover the painful region [42, 43]; however, the precise technical conditions for optimal application of the procedure remain a matter of debate [8], and the same applies to the proportion of patients successfully managed with SCS [44]. In this

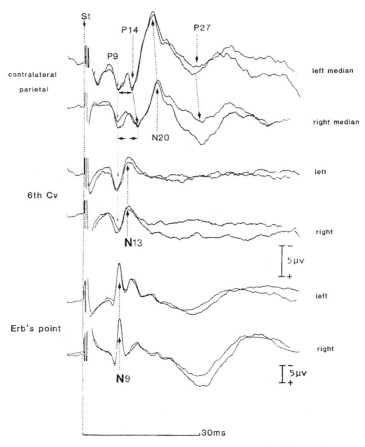

Fig. 1. Somatosensory evoked potentials (SEPs) after left and right median nerve stimulation, showing abnormal conduction time in the left dorsal column at the cervical level, reflected by unilateral increase of the P9-P14 interval. Peripheral (N9) and dorsal horn spinal responses (N13) are normal and symmetrical. This kind of minor abnormality does not entail severe lemniscus deafferentation and is associated with a good probability of success of spinal cord stimulation

context, the neurophysiological assessment of SCS is clinically relevant, first, in the preoperative period to document the functional integrity of the dorsal columns (DC), and second, after SCS implantation to assess objectively its effects on the dorsal horn spinal circuitry.

Preoperative Assessment of SCS Candidates Using Evoked Potentials
Despite 'optimal' positioning and technical control of SCS, this procedure is not likely to produce adequate pain control if the dorsal column fibers that should be stimulated are not functional any more. This may occur in conditions causing

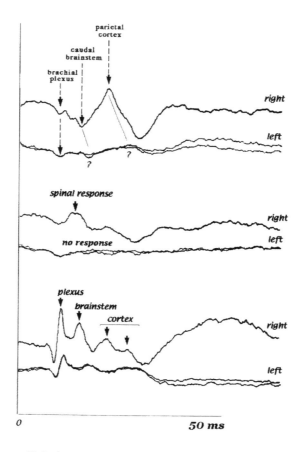

Fig. 2. SEPs in a case of left plexus traumatic injury. Stimulation of the preserved right side yielded normal peripheral, spinal, brainstem and cortical responses, while stimulation of the left side evoked a depressed peripheral (plexus) response with normal latency, indicating preservation of peripheral conduction but with some axonal loss. The absence of spinal response to left side stimulation (middle traces), associated with delay and desynchronisation of brainstem and cortical potentials suggests extensive injury at or proximal to the dorsal ganglion, and consequently ascending degeneration of dorsal column fibers. Such SEP pattern is associated with poor efficacy of spinal stimulation

destruction of dorsal ganglion cells (e.g. herpes zoster), or interrupting primary afferents between the ganglion and the dorsal root entry zone (radicular avulsion). In these cases the ascending fibers, disconnected from their soma in the dorsal ganglion, will undergo rapid degeneration up to their synapse in the lower medullary nuclei. The same may occur in case of intrinsic lesions of the cord white matter, such as spinal injury or multiple sclerosis, interrupting fibers within the dorsal columns. In all these cases the recording of SEPs permits us to assess the permeability of the DC/lemniscal system, and, in case of alteration, allows an estimation of the percentage of surviving functional fibers based on SEP amplitude. SEP features also help to locate topographically a plexus lesion proximal or distal to the dorsal ganglion, and thus are important to determine whether clinical anaesthesia/hypesthesia is likely to be associated or not with degeneration of DC fibers. It has been shown that clinical failure of SCS, including in instances of so-called "malposition", may be simply attributed to inadequate assessment of DC degeneration [45]. Also, the proportion of cases with good clinical efficacy has been shown to increase if a strict selection of patients is performed on the basis of DC functionality assessed with SEPs [45, 46]. Figures 1 and 2 illustrate different SEP patterns encountered in patients with neuropathic pain considered for possible spinal stimulation, which are associated with different probabilities of successful pain relief under neurostimulation.

The functional state of ascending spinothalamic pathways may now be assessed using laser-evoked responses; however, their impact on the patient's management during the pre-operative phases is not yet known, mainly because we do not know the possible importance for SCS success of preserved spinothalamic transmission. The main use of laser-evoked potentials (LEPs) in patients is, for the time being, to demonstrate the neuropathic nature of pain in patients refractory to pharmaco-

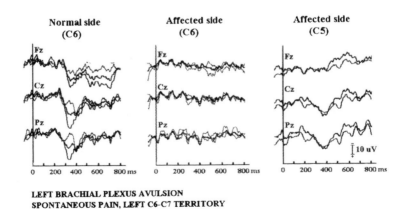

Fig. 3. Laser evoked potentials (LEPs) in a case of upper limb pain after plexus lesion. The neuropathic nature of the pain is substantiated by the severe alterations of LEPs to stimulation of the affected territory (C6), demonstrating significant loss of A-delta fibers from that territory. Note the persistence of normal LEPs after stimulation of a contiguous dermatome (C5) in the affected limb, suggesting restriction of axonal loss to the C6 spinal root

logical procedures. Thus, abnormally increased pain (especially if stimulation-related) on the background of reduced LEPs substantiates the neuropathic nature of the pain [47], while normal or enhanced LEPs to stimulation of a painful territory suggest the integrity of pain pathways and do not support the diagnosis of neuropathic pain (Fig. 3).

Assessment of SCS Efficacy with Nociceptive Reflexes
The neurophysiological effects of large fiber stimulation on spinal nociceptive transmission have been repeatedly demonstrated in animal models [2, 3, 48, 49]. However, the question whether equivalent effects are also active in human patients during SCS or TENS has remained debatable for many years – and to some extent even today. The existence of a superimposed psychological (placebo) effect [50] and the natural tendency to exaggerate past pain [51] greatly hamper the objective evaluation of SCS or TENS effects in individual patients. Gathering evidence of objective modifications on spinal or cortical responses to noxious stimuli during SCS is therefore important for the clinical evaluation of implanted patients, especially in cases of difficult control, or alleged inefficacy of the procedure after a satisfactory period.

Recording of nociceptive responses during SCS or TENS aims at demonstrating stimulation-related depression of the RIII reflex associated with pain relief. Reversible attenuation of nociceptive responses during SCS and TENS has indeed been evidenced in man [52-54, and Fig. 4] in a very similar fashion to that described by unit recordings in animals [2, 3, 48, 49], providing evidence of a neurophysiological effect of the procedure on the human spinal nociceptive circuitry.

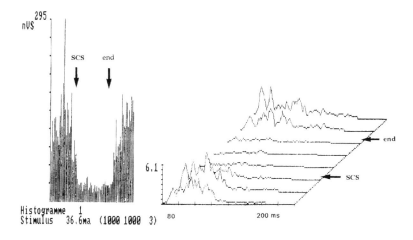

Fig. 4. Nociceptive reflexes during spinal cord stimulation (SCS) in man. Surface histograms in left side and averaged responses in the right side of the figure. The example illustrates rapid attenuation of nociceptive RIII reflexes after SCS onset, with rapid and complete reversion on SCS discontinuation. This pattern of nociceptive reflex behaviour is associated with good clinical efficacy of SCS. Reproduced from [53] by permission

Attenuation of spinal responses to acutely induced pain is consistent with pain detection decrease during neurostimulation [e.g. 55]. Moreover, analgesic neurostimulation has proved to be able to reduce or abolish the nociceptive RIII reflex while leaving virtually unaffected other reflexes non-nociceptive in nature [54] which are subserved in part by the same motor units [21]. Hence we may conclude that (a) neurostimulation effects are quite selective upon the processing of nociceptive inputs at the spinal level, and (b) its action upon RIII is consistent with an effect at the dorsal horn, rather than upon the motor branch of the response.

SCS-induced RIII depression has been found to be associated with good clinical efficacy of the procedure at short and middle term [26, 54]. Also, patients in whom AN induces an enhancement of nociceptive reflexes often report worsening of pain during neurostimulation – a paradoxical effect that has been documented clinically [56]. These observations suggest that RIII depression may be a good indicator of the pain-relieving effects of SCS. Considering that neurogenic pain is thought to depend in part on hyperexcitability of nociceptive dorsal horn neurons, and that RIII attenuation reflects depression of spinal nociceptive units, it is not surprising to find an association between RIII attenuation during SCS and pain relief. However, the link between RIII attenuation and pain relief is not straightforward: while RIII depression usually reverses shortly (Fig. 4) clinical relief may last for hours after SCS discontinuation. Therefore, transient RIII attenuation during SCS might be the human counterpart of nociceptive unit depression in the experimental animal, and other mechanisms, probably neurochemical, should be responsible for prolongation of clinical effects beyond the period of reflex suppression.

Dazinger et al. [57] have recently reproduced the depressive and rapidly reversible effects of non-noxious TENS on the segmental nociceptive RIII. More important, they have equally shown that *noxious* TENS (by use of piezo-electric currents) may exert a powerful and long-lasting depressive effect on the RIII, suggesting the action of a descending inhibitory system triggered by noxious stimuli and previously described in animals and man under the label "Diffuse noxious inhibitory control" (DNIC) [58]. These results may be important for the future application of neuromodulation procedures, inasmuch as the combination of segmental/non-noxious with heterotopic/noxious stimulations might be a useful alternative for pain control in cases refractory to conventional SCS (see 59 for a review).

Correlation of RIII changes and long term SCS efficacy remains unknown. A preliminary report has suggested a possible association between RIII results shortly after operation and clinical efficacy at 1-2 years follow-up [60], but this should be confirmed in larger, prospective studies. A general difficulty of this kind of study is that loss of SCS efficacy over time may be due to a number of technical or medical problems unpredictable at the time of RIII evaluation.

In summary, the recording of nociceptive RIII is non-invasive and safely applicable in clinical context. RIII recordings during neurostimulation procedures can be used (a) to select 'optimal' parameters of stimulation (in terms of the ability of the procedure to depress nociceptive reflexes); (b) to disclose presumed placebo effects; (c) to confirm the absence of neurophysiological effect in patients complaining of loss of efficacy, and (d) in general terms every time that an objective evaluation of stimulation effects upon nociceptive spinal circuitry is sought.

Assessment of SCS with Evoked Potentials

Somatosensory evoked potentials have shown attenuation of brainstem and cortical responses during TENS, without any change of peripheral potentials [61, 62]. This shows that TENS not only modifies the central transmission of nociceptive inputs, but also that of innocuous ascending information. The locus of interference between TENS and non-noxious somatosensory inputs appeared to be the cuneate nucleus, without significant effects on spinal intrinsic responses, thus suggesting that TENS does not influence the spinal integration of non-nociceptive information. This is at variance with studies during skin vibration, a stimulus strongly reminding of TENS, which has been shown to interfere strongly with innocuous somatic inputs both at brainstem and dorsal horn spinal level [63].

The effect of high-rate (TENS-like) vibration on cortical responses has been also studied using cortical evoked potentials to noxious laser stimuli (LEPs). Concurrently applied vibration (and also active movements of the fingers) increased pain threshold and reduced pain LEPs, thus reflecting pain inhibitory mechanisms set up by sensory inputs *via* large myelinated fibers. In contrast, continuous cooling decreased pain threshold, probably due to spatial summation of two kinds of nociceptive inputs mediated by the same pathways [64]. We are not aware of studies examining laser EPs during SCS or TENS in patients: since laser-EPs yield information on cortical responses only, the relative contribution of spinal and supraspinal mechansims to SCS-induced inhibition of pain inputs cannot be estimated by this technique alone. Animal models of neurogenic pain have recently suggested that inhibition of abnormally enhanced nociceptive reflexes by SCS is operative at spinal level, and does not necessarily involve supraspinal mechanisms [65]. However, the concomitant existence of supraspinal mechanisms in man cannot be ruled out, especially in view of the proved supraspinal effect of TENS in the brainstem somatosensory transduction (see above, 61, 63].

Assessment of SCS with Functional Imaging

PET imaging of changes in regional CBF has been attempted during spinal neurostimulation [38]. The results showed that SCS modulates regional cerebral blood flow in brain areas known to be associated with nociception and also with cardiovascular control, including the periaqueductal grey, orbitofrontal and cingulate cortices, the dorsomedial and posterior thalamus, and the temporal and insular gyri. Although it is too early to interpret, precisely these results, increasing amounts of data on brain responses during pain-relieving procedures, both pharmacological and non-pharmacological, should improve our understanding of the relationships between brain changes in cerebral blood flow and pain relief. For example, both opioid analgesia [66, 67] and neurostimulations for pain relief [38, 40, 68] tend to increase CBF in the orbitofrontal and anterior cingulate cortices (ACC), at very similar sites where blood flow has been found to be decreased in allodynic or chronic pain patients [69]. Although preliminary, these data suggest that regulation of activity at the orbitofrontal/ACC regions may play a role in stimulation-induced pain relief. This region contains a high density of opioid receptors [70], and part of the neurostimulation-related CBF changes might therefore depend on opioid receptor activation. Although no direct proof of this is currently available, it is likely that in vivo neuroreceptor mapping studies in future years will be of importance for the understanding of these issues and therefore for the treatment of chronic pain

Motor Cortex Stimulation for Intractable Pain
The use of motor cortex stimulation (MCS) for pain control was documented during the early 1990s by Tsubokawa et al. [13, 14]. These authors described a chronic MCS procedure which, in preliminary studies, provided satisfactory control of central post-stroke pain with a better risk/benefit ratio than stimulation of deeper structures such as the thalamus. Since then, the use of MCS for analgesic purposes is being increasingly used for both poststroke pain [19, 17] and other neuropathic conditions including trigeminal pain [15, 18] and central pain after Wallenberg's syndrome [16].

In spite of the encouraging results of MCS, the reasons accounting for its analgesic efficacy have not yet been elucidated, and its clinical application remains therefore largely empirical. In a recent study, Katayama et al. [16] observed that a high degree of corticospinal impairment could predict poor MCS efficacy, and the same group proposed that the efficacy rate of the procedure may benefit from pre-selection of patients according to their response to different analgesic drugs (morphine vs. barbiturates). In spite of these clinical insights, the mechanisms of action of MCS remains a mystery today. Tsubokawa et al. [14] have suggested that, in cases of thalamic pain, MCS is superior to thalamic stimulation due to its more rostral level of application, which ensures activation of preserved functional zones acting upon deafferented structures. Precentral gyrus stimulation could then entail analgesia through secondary activation of non-nociceptive neurons in the sensory cortex, via backward excitation of axons connecting somatosensory and motor areas. This hypothesis has been supported by histochemical changes within the primary sensory cortex of rats subject to chronic motor stimulation [71], but has not been confirmed in humans. On the other hand, experimental data also point to the thalamus as a possible target of MCS, since this procedure (unlike SI stimulation) was able to attenuate thalamic hyperactivity after spinothalamic transection in cats [72].

PET-Scan Studies during MCS
Whatever the mechanisms underlying MCS clinical effects, these are likely to be mediated by regional changes in synaptic activity – and thus of cerebral blood flow – which can be measured in humans using PET (see earlier section). Accordingly, during the past years we have conducted several PET studies to assess the regional CBF changes of patients undergoing MCS for central intractable pain. In preliminary studies on individual patients CBF was found to increase during MCS in the thalamus ipsilateral to stimulation, in the orbito-frontal and cingulate gyri and in the upper brainstem [40]. Further studies on groups of subjects with intractable pain of various etiologies (some of them still under evaluation) have confirmed the existence of significant CBF increases during MCS in the lateral and medial thalamus, the anterior cingulate/orbitofrontal cortex (BA32), the anterior insula/medial temporal lobe and the upper brainstem, near the periaqueductal grey [41] (Fig. 5). The thalamic areas undergoing maximally significant CBF changes were the ven-

tral-lateral and ventral-anterior nuclei, i.e. the thalamic regions directly connected with motor and premotor cortices. Conversely, no significant CBF changes appeared in primary motor or somatic areas during the procedure. These results are taken as evidence that descending axons, rather than apical dendrites, are primarily activated by MCS, and highlight the thalamus as the key structure mediating functional MCS effects.

A model of MCS action may therefore be proposed, whereby activation of thalamic nuclei connected with motor and premotor cortices is a necessary (although not sufficient) step allowing the pain-relieving activity of this procedure. Thalamic activation, which is a common effect of pain relieving procedures [73, 74] would trigger a cascade of synaptic events influencing activity in other pain-related structures, including the anterior cingulate gyri, insula/MTL, subthalamic areas and upper brainstem. As a consequence, MCS could influence the affective-emotional component of chronic pain by way of cingulate/orbitofrontal effects, and lead to descending inhibition of pain impulses by activation of the brainstem. Among the cingulate subdivisions, the perigenual region bordering orbitofrontal cortex (BA32, i.e. that showing maximal changes to MCS) is considered to subserve in part the affective components of pain [75-77], and generally the processing of emotional stimuli [78]. Thus, the analgesic effects of MCS might partly derive from a transient blunting of the distressful reaction to pain, rather than from an actual decrease of its intensity. Since thalamic functional changes may need to reach a threshold in order to influence other structures, the lack of clinical effect might result in some instances from a failure to attain such threshold.

SEPs and Nociceptive Reflexes in the Assessment of MCS Mechanisms
In our experience, somatosensory responses from primary sensory cortex remain stable during MCS [41]: thus, the procedure does not appear to modify the general excitability of primary sensory cortex to external inputs. This is consistent with the absence of proven haemodynamic changes in primary sensory areas (see Fig. 5), although this result should be confirmed by further, higher resolution imaging studies. Recent, unpublished results suggest that cortical potentials evoked by painful heat (CO_2-laser stimulation) might be depressed during MCS in selected patients [79], this result being reminding of the pain-SEP attenuation observed during peripheral vibration or limb movement [64]. Pain SEPs to laser stimuli have been shown to be composed of an early, lateralised response probably originating in second somatic areas, followed by a vertex complex of multiple generators, including the anterior cingulate, insular and/or medial temporal cortices [80-83]. The first response has been related to sensory aspects of pain processing, while the second is modulated by attentional and cognitive factors; hence, if the effects of MCS (or other neuromodulating procedures) on pain SEPs are confirmed, it will be important to determine their relative repercussion on each of these functional response subdivisions.

MCS may also lead to descending inhibition of pain impulses at the dorsal horn level. This putative mechanism of MCS-induced analgesia was already postulated by Adams et al. [12], who considered that activation of corticospinal axons was able to inhibit nociceptive neurons at the spinal level. We have observed changes in

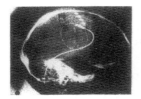
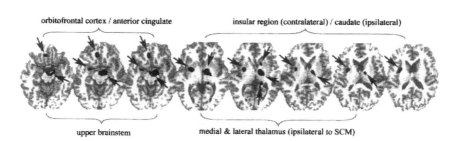

Fig. 5. Brain regions which showed significant increase of blood flow during motor cortex stimulation (MCS) in the study by Garcia-Larrea et al. (1999). Pooled results from 9 subjects. The region with maximally significant flow increases during stimulation was the thalamus ipsilateral, but significant increases were also observed in subthalamic and brainstem regions, anterior (perigenual) cingulate gyri, insula, caudate and putamen. Conversely, no significant changes in blood flow were observed in primary sensory or motor areas (not shown in the figure)

spinal nociceptive reflexes during cortical stimulation [41], analogous to those previously described during SCS (see above). Descending inhibition triggered by cortical stimulation might explain the efficacy of the procedure upon the 'evoked components' of pain (i.e. allodynia, hyperalgesia and hyperpathia). Early investigators noted that stimulation of central motor fibers may inhibit afferent transmission in the dorsal horn [10, 11], an effect that might be at the basis of flexion reflex attenuation in patients submitted to MCS.

Conclusion

In well-established neurostimulation procedures the preoperative recording of SEPs improves patient selection by determining the functional state of the dorsal column system, while the postoperative assessment with nociceptive reflexes yields objective data on the effects on the spinal circuitry. In new and promising neuromodulation schemes such as MCS, the mechanisms of which are not yet understood, the combination of clinical electrophysiology and functional neuroimaging provides insight into the possible mechanisms of action, guides clinical research and may in the future contribute to a better selection of patients.

References

1. Melzack R, Wall P (1965) Pain mechanisms: a new theory. Science 150:971-97
2. Handwerker HO, Iggo A, Zimmermann M (1975) Segmental and supraspinal actions on dorsal horn neurons responding to noxious and non-noxious skin stimuli. Pain 1:147-165
3. Lindblom U, Tapper N, Wiesenfeld Z (1977) The effect of dorsal column stimulation on the nociceptive response of dorsal horn cells and its relevance for pain suppression. Pain 4:133-144
4. Gerhart KD, Yezierski RP, Fang ZR, Willis WD (1983) Inhibition of primate spinothalamic tract neurons by stimulation in ventral posterior lateral thalamic nucleus. Possible mechanisms. J. Neurophysiol 49:406-423
5. Wall PD (1978) The gate-control theory of pain mechanisms. Brain 101:1-18
6. Meyerson BA (1983) Electrostimulation procedures: effects, presumed rationale, and possible mechanisms. In Bonica JL, Ed. Advances in Pain Research and Therapy. Vol. 5, New York, Raven Press pp 495-534
7. Gybels J, Kuypers R (1995) Subcortical stimulation in humans and pain. In: Desmedt JE, Bromm B, (ed) Advances in Pain Research and Therapy n°22 (Pain and the Brain), Basel, Karger pp 187-199
8. Holsheimer J (1997) Effectiveness of spinal cord stimulation in the management of chronic pain: analysis of technical drawbacks and solutions. Neurosurgery 1997 40:990-996
9. Jessurun GAJ, Dejongste MJL, Blanksma PK (1996) Current views on neurostimulation in the treatment of cardiac ischemic syndromes. Pain 66:109-116
10. Lindblom U, Ottosson JO (1957) Influence of pyramidal stimulation upon the relay of coarse cutaneous afferents in the dorsal horn. Acta Physiol Scand 38:309-318
11. Andersen P, Eccles JC, Sears TA (1962) Presynaptic inhibitory action of cerebral cortex on the spinal cord. Nature194:740-741
12. Adams JE, Hosobuchi Y, Fields HL (1974) Stimulation of internal capsule for relief of chronic pain. J Neurosurg 41:740-744
13. Tsubokawa T, Katayama Y, Yamamoto T et al (1991) Chronic motor cortex stimulation for the treatment of central pain. Acta Neurochir (Suppl 52):137-139
14. Tsubokawa T, Katayama Y, Yamamoto T et al (1993a) Chronic motor cortex stimulation in patients with thalamic pain. J Neurosurg 78:393-401
15. Meyerson BA, Lindblom U, Linderoth B et al (1993) Motor cortex stimulation as a treatment of trigeminal neuropathic pain. Acta Neurochirurg (suppl. 58): 150-153
16. Katayama Y, Tsubokawa T, Yamamoto T (1994) Chronic motor cortex stimulation for central deafferentation pain: experience with bulbar pain secondary to Wallenberg syndrome. Stereotact Funct Neurosurg 62:295-299
17. Katayama Y, Fukaya C, Yamamoto T (1998) Poststroke pain control by chronic motor stimulation: neurological characteristics predicting a favorable response. J Neurosurg 89:585-591
18. Ebel H, Rust D, Tronnier V et al (1996) Chronic precentral stimulation in trigeminal neuropathic pain. Acta Neurochir 138:1300-1306
19. Herregodts P, Stadnik T, Deridder F, Dhaens J (1996) Cortical stimulation for central neuropathic pain: 3-D surface MRI for easy determination of the motor cortex. In: Adv Stereotact Funct Neurosurg 11:132-135
20. Sherrington CS (1910) Flexion-reflex of the limb, crossed extension-reflex, and reflex stepping and standing. J Physiol (Lond.) 40:28-121
21. Hugon M (1973) Exteroceptive reflexes to stimulation of the sural nerve in normal man. In: New Developments in Electromyography and Clinical Neurophysiology, Vol. III, JE Desmedt (ed) Basel, Karger:713-729

22. Willer JC (1977) Comparative study of perceived pain and nociceptive flexion reflex in man. Pain 3:69-80
23. Willer JC (1984) Nociceptive flexion reflex as a physiological correlate of pain sensation in humans. Handbook of Physiology, Amsterdam, Elsevier pp 87-110
24. Duggan AW, Foong FW (1985) Bicuculline and spinal inhibition produced by dorsal column stimulation in the cat. Pain 22:249-259
25. Carstens E, Campbell IG (1988) Parametric and pharmacological studies of midbrain supression of the hind limb flexion withdrawal reflex in the rat. Pain, 33:201-213
26. García-Larrea L., Mauguière F (1990) Electrophysiological assessment of nociception in normals and patients: the use of nociceptive spinal reflexes. Electroencephal Clin Neurophysiol (Suppl. 41):102-118
27. Bathien N (1971) Réflexes spinaux chez l'Homme et niveaux d'attention. Electroenceph clin Neurophysiol 30:32-37
28. Willer JC, Boureau F, Albe-Fessard D (1979) Supraspinal influences on nociceptive flexion reflexes and pain sensation in man. Brain Res 179:61-68
29. Willer JC, Albe-Fessard D (1980) Electrophysiological evidence for a release of endogenous opiates in stress-induced 'analgesia' in man. Brain Res 198:419-426
30. García-Larrea L, Charles N, Sindou M, Mauguière F (1993) Flexion reflexes following alterolateral cordotomy in man: dissociation between subjective pain and nociceptive reflex RIII. Pain 55:139-149
31. Mauguière F (1995) Description and origins of SEP components. In: Binnie C et al. (eds) Clinical Neurophysiology, Vol. 1. Oxford, Butterworth - Heinemann: 393-421
32. Bromm B, Treede RD (1991) Laser-evoked cerebral potentials in the assessment of cutaneous pain sensitivity in normal subjects and patients. Rev Neurol 147: 625-643
33. Arendt-Nielsen L (1991) Characteristics, detection and modulation of laser-evoked vertex potentials. Acta Anaesthesiol. Scandinavica 38 (suppl. 101): 1-44
34. García-Larrea L, Peyron R, Laurent B, Mauguière F (1997) Association and dissociation between laser-evoked potentials and pain sensation. Neuroreport 8:3785-3789
35. Fox PT, Mintun MA (1989) Noninvasive functional brain mapping by change-distribution analysis of averaged PET images of H2150 tissue activity. J Nucl Med 30:141-149
36. Sokoloff L, Porter A, Roland P, et al (1991) General Discussion. In: Chadwick C, Derek J, Whelan J (eds) Exploring brain functional anatomy with positron emission tomography; Ciba Foundation Symposium n°163, London, Wiley & Sons: 43-56
37. Peyron R, Laurent B, García-Larrea L (2000) Functional imaging of pain: A review and meta-analysis. Neurophysiol. Clin 30:263-288
38. Hautvast RWM, Terhorst GJ, Dejong BM, et al (1997) Relative changes in regional cerebral blood flow during spinal cord stimulation in patients with refractory angina pectoris. Eur Journal Neurosci 9:1178-1183
39. Katayama Y, Tsubokawa T, Hirayama T (1986) Response of regional cerebral blood flow and oxygen metabolism to thalamic stimulation in humans as revealed by positron emission tomography. J Cereb Blood Flow Metab 6:637-641
40. Peyron R, García-Larrea L, Deiber MP et al (1995) Electrical stimulation of precentral cortical area in the treatment of central pain: electrophysiological and PET study. Pain 62:275-286
41. García-Larrea L, Peyron R, Mertens P, et al (1999). Electrical stimulation of motor cortex for pain control: a combined PET-scan and electrophysiological study. Pain 83:259-273
42. Barolat G, Zeme S, Ketcik B (1991) Multifactorial analysis of epidural spinal cord stimulation. Stereotact Funct Neurosurg 56:77-103
43. North RB (1993). Spinal cord stimulation for chronic, intractable pain. In: Devinsky O, Beric A, Dogali M (eds) Electrical and Magnetic Stimulation of the Brain and Spinal Cord. New York, Raven Press:289-301

44. Segal R, Stacey BR, Rudy TE et al (1998) Spinal cord stimulation revisited. Neurol. Res 20:391-396
45. Keravel Y, Sindou M, Blond S (1991) Stimulation and ablative neurosurgical procedures in the peripheral nerves and the spinal cord for deafferentation and neuropathic pain. In: Besson JM, Guilbaud G (eds) Lesions of Primary Afferent Fibers as a Tool for the Study of Clinical Pain. Amsterdam, Elsevier:315-334
46. Mertens P, Sindou M, Gharios B et al (1992) Spinal cord stimulation for pain treatment: prognostic value of somesthetic evoked potentials. Acta Neurochir (Wien) 117:90-91
47. Wu Q, Garcia-Larrea L, Mertens P et al (1999) Hyperalgesia with loss of laser EPs in neuropathic pain. Pain 80:209-214
48. Hillman P, Wall PD (1969) Inhibitory and excitatory factors influencing the receptive fields of lamina V spinal cord cells. Exp Brain Res 9:284-306
49. Brown AG, Hamann WC, Martin HF (1973) Interactions of cutaneous myelinated (A) and non myelinated (C) fibers on transmission through the spinocervical tract. Brain Res 53:222-226
50. Marchand S, Charest J, Li J et al (1993) Is TENS purely a placebo effect? A controlled study on chronic low back pain. Pain 54:99-106
51. Erskine A, Morley S, Pearce S (1990) Memory for pain: a review. Pain 41:255-265
52. Boureau F, Keravel Y, Hugenard P (1981) Effects of dorsal column stimulation on human spinal reflexes. Preliminary results. Pain (Suppl 1): 319
53. García-Larrea L, Sindou M, Mauguière F (1989) Clinical use of nociceptive flexor reflex recording in functional neurosurgical procedures. Acta Neurochir Suppl (Wien) 46:53-57
54. García-Larrea L, Sindou M, Mauguière F (1989) Nociceptive flexion reflexes during analgesic neurostimulation in man. Pain 39:145-156
55. Marchand S, Bushnell MC, Molina-Negro P et al (1991) The effects of dorsal column stimulation on measures of clinical and experimental pain in man. Pain 45:249-257
56. Cole JD, Illis LS, Sedwick EM (1987) Pain produced by spinal cord stimulation in a patient with allodynia and pseudo-tabes. J Neurol Neurosurg Psychiat 50:1083-1084
57. Dazinger N, Rozenberg S, Bourgeois P et al (1998) Depressive effects of segmental and heterotopic application of transcutaneous electrical nerve stimulation and piezo-electric current on lower limb nociceptive reflex in human subjects. Arch Phys Med Rehabil 79:191-200
58. Le Bars D, Dickenson AH, Besson J-M (1979) Diffuse noxious inhibitory controls: Effects on dorsal horn convergent neurons in the rat. Pain 6:283-304
59. Willer JC, Boussahira D, Le Bars D (1979). Bases neurophysiologiques du phénomène de contre-irritation: les contrôles inhibiteurs induits par stimulations nociceptives. Neurophysiol. Clin 29:379-400
60. Parise M, García-Larrea L, Mertens P, Sindou M (1998) A estimulaçao medular no tratamento da dor crônica. Presentation to the XXII Brazilian Congress of Neurosurgery, Rio de Janeiro, 4-11 Sept. Book of Abstracts, pp 412
61. Nardone A, Schieppati M (1989) Influences of transcutaneous electrical stimulation of cutaneous and mixed nerves on subcortical and cortical somatosensory evoked potentials. Electroencephal clin Neurophysiol 74:24-35
62. Urasaki E, Wada S, Yasukouchi H, Yokota A (1998) Effect of transcutaneous electrical nerve stimulation (TENS) on central nervous system amplification of somatosensory input. J Neurol 245:143-148
63. Ibañez V, Deiber MP, Mauguière F (1989) Interference of vibrations with input transmission in dorsal horn and cuneate nucleus in man: a study of somatosensory evoked potentials (SEPs) to electrical stimulation of median nerve and fingers. Exp Brain Res 75:599-610

64. Kakigi R, Shibasaki H (1992) Mechanisms of pain relief by vibration and movement. J Neurol Neurosurg Psychiatr 55:282-286
65. Ren B, Linderoth B, Meyerson BA (1996) Effects of spinal cord stimulation on the flexor reflex and involvement of supraspinal mechanisms: An experimental study in mononeuropathic rats. J Neurosurg 84:244-249
66. Firestone LL, Gyulai F, Mintun M et al (1996) Human brain activity response to fentanyl imaged by positron emission tomography, Anesth Analg 82:1247-51
67. Adler LJ, Gyulai FE, Diehl DJ, et al (1997), Regional brain activity changes associated with fentanyl analgesia elucidated by positron emission tomography. Anesth Analg 84:120-126
68. Duncan G., Kupers RC, Marchand S, et al (1998) Stimulation of human thalamus for pain relief: possible modulatory circuits revealed by Positron Emission Tomography. J. Neurophysiol 80:3326-3330
69. Peyron R, García-Larrea L, Grégoire MC, et al (1998) Allodynia after lateral-medullary (Wallenberg) infarct. A Positron Emission Tomography (PET) study, Brain 121:345-356
70. Jones AKP, Qi LY, Fujirawa T et al (1991) In vivo distribution of opioid receptors in man in relation to the cortical projections of the medial and lateral pain systems measured with positron emission tomography, Neurosci Lett 126:25-28
71. Tsubokawa T, Katayama Y, Yamamoto T, et al (1993b) Treatment of deafferentation pain with thalamic and motor cortex stimulation: possible role of reorganization of neural circuits. VIIth World Congress on Pain. Book of Abstracts, IASP Publications, Seattle:504-505
72. Hirayama T, Tsubokawa T, Katayama Y, et al (1990) Tonic changes in activity of thalamic lemniscal relay neurons following spino-thalamic tractotomy in cats: effects of motor cortex stimulation. Pain; (suppl. 5):S273
73. Di Piero V, Jones AKP, Iannotti F, et al (1991) Chronic pain: a PET study of the central effects of percutaneous high cervical cordotomy. Pain, 46:9-12
74. Pagni CA, Canavero S (1995) Functional thalamic depression in a case of reversible central pain due to a spinal intramedullary cyst. Case report. J Neurosurg 83:163-165
75. Foltz EL, White LE (1962) Pain 'relief' by frontal cingulumotomy. J Neurosurg 19:89-100
76. Vogt B, Finch DM, Olson C (1992) Functional heterogeneity in cingulate cortex: The anterior executive and posterior evaluative regions. Cerebral Cortex 2:435-443
77. Devinsky O, Morrell MJ, Vogt BA (1995) Contributions of the anterior cingulate cortex to behaviour. Brain, 118:279-306
78. Lane RD, Fink GR, Chau PML, Dolan RJ (1997) Neural activation during selective attention to subjective emotional responses. Neuroreport, 8:3969-3972
79. Nuti C (1998) La stimulation antalgique du cortex precentral. Synthèse des données actuelles. Unpublished MD Thesis, University of St Étienne, France:150pp
80. Bromm B, Chen ACN (1995) Brain electrical source analysis of laser evoked potentials in response to painful trigeminal nerve stimulation. Electroenceph clin Neurophysiol 95:14-26
81. Valeriani M, Rambaud L, Mauguière F (1996) Scalp topography and dipolar source modelling of potentials evoked by CO_2 laser stimulation of the hand, Electroencephal clin Neurophysiol 100:343-353
82. García-Larrea L (1998) Multimodal approaches to generators of laser evoked potentials: with a little help from our friends. Pain Forum 7:216-220
83. Frot M, Mauguière F (1999) Les réponses operculo-insulaires aux stimulations cutanées nociceptives chez l'Homme. Neurophysiol Clin 29:401-410

Chapter 10

Acute Postoperative Pain Service Models

G. Galimberti, P. Di Marco, A. Conti

After surgery, patients frequently experience severe pain, and a significant portion receives less than adequate analgesia [1, 2]. Furthermore, surveys in 1980s showed that as many as 30-75% of patients still receive inadequate pain treatment in the postoperative period, despite an increasing awareness of this issue [3-6].

It is remarkable that Smith [7], in an editorial, asserted "what is so surprising is that, this deplorable state of affairs has persisted and continues to persist in many hospitals, despite considerable advances in the pharmacology of analgesic drugs and description of new and improved methods of relieving pain". However, although recent years have seen the widespread use of modern and effective analgesic techniques, such as epidural analgesia, postoperative regional blocks, and patient-controlled analgesia (PCA) for the relief of postoperative pain, the most frequently used technique in surgical wards still remains the use of intra-muscolar opioids prescribed by ward surgeon and administered by ward nurse on an as-needed basis [8]. The continuous insult of nociceptive stimuli during the postoperative period may be harmful and deleterious for the patient's outcome [9, 10], and it is becoming clear that the solution of the problem of the postoperative pain lies in the development of an organization to exploit existing expertise [11]. Currently, the implementation of the acute postoperative pain services (APS) in hospitals is strongly recommended by a committee of experts and its role in the management of the quality of postoperative pain relief is increasing year by year.

Management of Postoperative Acute Pain

Clinical Implications

Pain is a complex experience, including physiological, psychological, and experiential aspects, which together account for the sensation of pain. According to the definition of pain adopted by the International Association for Study of Pain, we might define pain as "a subjective and emotional experience associated with actual or potential tissue damage or expressed in terms of such damage". It is obvious that visual analogic scales (VAS) are a very useful tool to evaluate the pain intensity but cannot express the multiple aspects related to the pain experience. The beginning of nociception is generated by nociceptors widely distributed throughout the body, and the signals are then transferred by afferent sensory nerve fibers to the spinal cord and then to the brain. The inflammatory response, resulting from trauma damage due to the surgical intervention, is able to unleash and successively amplify a strong and important neurotransmitter cascade. It is well recognized that adequate pain relief reduces complications and mortality after major surgery, increasing pulmonary function, chest expansion, effective cough effort, and cooperation with the chest physiotherapist [10, 12]. Also adequate analgesia reduces sympathetic activity, which causes tachycardia, hypertension, increased stroke volume, cardiac work and myocardial oxygen consumption. The risk of myocardial ischemia or infarction is reduced, as is the risk of deep vein thrombosis in patients at rest, with platelet aggregation and venous stasis. Furthermore, the recent popularity of the fast-tracking anesthesia programs and the increasing number and complexity of day-surgery procedures have increased the need for optimal pain relief. Inadequate analgesia is a major cause of delayed discharge [13-15].

Consequently, postoperative pain is dangerous not only because it is a potent trigger for the stress response, having adverse effects on various organ systems, but also because it may determine spinal cord hyperexcitability – the so-called wind-up phenomenon – responsible itself for hyperalgesic and/or spontaneous painful syndromes [16-19]. The "wind-up" mechanism seems to be able to modify the physiological and anatomical neuronal characteristics, through a mechanism called spinal cord "neuroplasticity" and, even though the physiopathology is not yet fully understood, it constitutes a sort of neurochemical memory of the pain. In any event, a great contribution to this seems to be intracellular transduction of extracellular signals, involving a cascade of phosphorylation-dephosphorylation events leading to modulation of the activity of several different molecules. Repeated nociceptive stimulation determines the release of a variety of excitatory neurotransmitters, such as amino acids glutamate and aspartate, activating N-methyl-d-aspartate (NMDA) and α-amino-3-hydroxy-5-methyl-4-isoxazoleproprionate (AMPA) receptors located in dorsal horn neurones [20, 21]. NMDA receptors, in particular, induce the release of substance P and neurokinin A, maintaining the spinal hypersensitivity and potentiating the transmission of nociceptive messages [22]. As a consequence of this receptor activation, there is an increased gene expression from some postsynaptic neurones. The c-*fos* and c-*jun* proto-oncogenes, for example, are part of this cellular program that guarantees synaptic plasticity, i.e., the capacity of neurones to modify their synapsis with activity and experience [23]. This activation of transcription factors by synaptic activity might represent the possible link between neurothrophin and neuroplasticity in the developing, as well as the central nervous systems. Consequently, the appearance of new antigenys in spinal cord neurones, as a phenotypic expression of the proto-oncogenes c-*fos* and c-*jun*, could be the first sign of a structural and chronic modification of protein synthesis providing a persistent track of pain suffered.

Multimodal Approach

Since the development of balanced anesthesia, it is clear that in anesthesia and analgesia, it is better to use more drugs together, with different mechanisms of action than to use only one. This synergistic interaction of drugs increases the effectiveness and safety of the treatment. The gains from drug and technique combination are twofold, reducing the drug dose and, therefore, the side effects. If the mechanism of action is completely separate and the side effects of the drugs and techniques are quite different, it is possible to reduce the total drug dose and, therefore, the incidence and severity of the side effects. Moreover, in the presence of synergism, the final effects are more than simply additive [24]. Thus, at present most anesthesia and analgesia techniques, particularly with high-risk patients, have a multimodal approach in order to reduce afferent input to the spinal cord, to block the autonomic response, and to avoid the stress response to surgery. Consequently a multimodal approach to postoperative acute pain includes wound infiltration [25-28], pre-emptive analgesia [29-35], peripheral regional blocks, the use of common analgesic protocols, the routine assessment of pain intensity at the bedside, and regular audit and staff education.

Organizational Factors: the APS

A task force of experts from Australia, United Kingdom, and United States recommends the implementation of APS as a major means of improving the quality of postoperative pain relief. Moreover, several interdisciplinary committees of experts have published guidelines that recommend frequent bedside pain assessment, evaluation of treatment efficacy, and a collaborative interdisciplinary organization for postoperative pain relief [36-38].

The idea of a service dedicated to relieve acute postoperative pain was first introduced in Germany in 1985 [39], but the first description of APS was published in 1988 by Ready et al. [40]. In the United States, the development of APS proceeded at a remarkable rate so that, currently, all major institutions in the United States have APS. In Europe, the situation is quite different. In some countries such as the United Kingdom [41], Sweden, and Holland the concept of APS has been widely accepted, and dedicated pain services have been established in many locations. In other countries, most hospitals are inadequate for the management of postoperative pain, and thus treatment continues to be inadequate. In 1990 a report by a joint working party of the Royal College of Surgeons and College of Anaesthesists was published, as an attempt to establish APS in all major hospital in the United Kingdom [42]. Within 4 years the percentage of hospitals in the United Kingdom with some sort of APS increased from 2.8 to 42.7%; the percentage of hospitals with at least one physician attending to acute pain management increased from 5,7 to 65.2%, while the percentage of hospitals with a dedicated acute pain nurse increased from 2.3 to 39.3%. There was also a significant increase in educational programs for medical and nursing staff about pain relief, and an increase in protocols and guidelines [43]. The main targets of these APS are the frequent pain evaluation by VAS, checking the analgesic treatment, and documentation of pain relief at the bedside of the patient. There is still strong debate about which APS organization is the best, in particular to restrict costs. In the literature, several models of APSs are described.

At present, the main models are the anesthesiologist-based APS proposed by

Ready et al. [40] and used in United States, and the nurse-based anesthesiologist-supervised APS proposed in Sweden by Rawal [6].

Anesthesiologist-Based APS [40]

Why an anesthesiologist-based system? Because anesthesiologists are familiar with the use of larger amounts of strong opioids, even over a prolonged period of time, with fewer side effects or respiratory depression, and are able to treat their complications and side effects [44]. Pain management is an unquestionable part of the care of patients in the postoperative period [45]. Additionally, seeing the results of decisions made by colleagues in the operating room has a significant educational value for the APS anaesthetist and could be used for assessment of the quality of care. Finally, alterations to prescriptions outside of standard protocol require a doctor [46].

APS staff includes several figures: staff anesthesiologists, and resident anesthesiologists or pain fellows, specially trained nurses and pharmacists, and physiotherapists or psychologists in some institutions [47]. Daily activity of APS includes clinical management of postoperative pain, consultation for postoperative pain management, informal education of ward nurses and medical and surgical house staff, and assisting operating room anesthesiologists in planning analgesic care for their patients.

Surgeons identify the patients who require the consultation of the anesthesiology team to consider the possibility of postoperative pain management. The possibilities are discussed jointly with patients during the routine preoperative visit. However, before implementation, the recommended plan for postoperative pain management is discussed with the surgeon to confirm its suitability. Surgeons also establish oral analgesic prescriptions to become effective when primary analgesia is discontinued: this facilitates a smooth transition.

The three main techniques used by anesthesiologists for the control of pain in the perioperative setting are:
1. PCA – with or without basal infusion – with systemic opioids;
2. epidural analgesia (EA) with opioids or opioid/local anesthetic mixture (or intratechal opiods);
3. regional anesthesia (RA) techniques, including (but not limited to) inter-costal blocks, plexus infusions, and pre- or postincisional wound infiltration by local anesthetics [48-50].

Specially trained and certified nurses can provide for pump refilling with narcotic or anesthetic drugs into epidural catheters, and this makes the use of this form of analgesia easier to be managed.

The service provides a 24-h coverage. Clinical rounds on all patients receiving PCA or EA are made each morning by the entire staff. Out of regular working hours, services are provided by a pain fellow or senior anesthesiology resident on an on-call basis.

In the PCA group vital signs and sedation level are monitored every 2 h for the first 8 h; every 4 h thereafter. In the EA group, ventilation and respiratory rate are assessed hourly for the first 24 h. After the 1st day, only sedation level is monitored hourly. In both groups, the duration of monitoring is 48 h.

Nurse-Based Anesthesiologist-Supervised APS [6]

The key-points of this model are: regular recording of pain intensity and treatment efficacy; use of regional anesthesia techniques only in appropriate patients; enrolment of every patient; use of protocols, standard orders, and guidelines for dose of analgesia, patient monitoring, and management of potential complications. On this basis, routine daily ward rounds and patient management do not require the physical involvement of the anesthesiologist and can be performed by a specially trained nurse.

The organization of APS includes several personnel: acute pain anesthesiologist, section anesthesiologist, "pain representative" ward-surgeon, "pain representative" day nurse and night nurse, acute pain nurse.

The modality of analgesia is decided preoperatively by the section anesthesiologist. Every patient is given at least 1 g paracetamol rectally or orally 4 times a day. During the preoperative visit, patients to undergo special techniques for pain management (PCA, EA or RA) are selected.

After surgical intervention VAS is measured by ward nurses, according to the modality of analgesia. Patient assessment in the postoperative period is performed every 3 h for the majority of patients, every hour in patients receiving PCA or EA, before and 45 min after treatment. Ward nurses have also the faculty to administer epidural opioids and local anesthetics and to set up PCA pumps. The VAS scores are recorded on the bedside vital sign chart, together with other vital signs such as temperature, pulse, and blood pressure. These values are checked by the acute pain nurse during her daily round of all surgical wards, who refers every problem to the section anesthesiologist.

The APS monitoring of the patient is stopped when VAS is lower than 3 without treatment on three consecutive measurements. Standard orders and guidelines regarding protocols of pain treatment, monitoring, and treatment of side effects are written for every ward in cooperation with the surgeons. Two "pain representative" day or night nurses are responsible for application of these protocols in the ward. The section anesthesiologist is responsible for postoperative pain in his ward, while a "pain representative" surgeon is responsible for pain management. An acute pain anesthesiologist coordinates all APSs of the hospitals and is responsible for in-service teaching activity. Other APS models are described in the literature.

Nurse-Controlled APS [51]

After surgical intervention, the patient is transferred to the recovery room, where he receives intravenous pethidine as required. When he leaves the recovery room, primary postoperative analgesia starts. The nurse prepares a solution by diluting

500 mg of pethidine in 500 ml physiological solution (standard dilution, 1 mg for 1 ml). Then, the solution is infused through a flow-guard infusion device. The nurse could titrate the infusion rate of opioid between 0 and 40 ml for 1 h, to achieve an adequate grade of analgesia as judged by the patient, without excessive grade of sedation. Whenever analgesia is insufficient with the rate of infusion previously set, a bolus injection of 20-40 ml of solution could be administered by the nurse to regain pain control.

Pain scores are measured hourly for 24 h using a verbal rating scale (VRS) from 0 to 10. Levels of nausea and sedation are measured hourly for 24 h. With this model there are no differences between pain level, frequency, and severity of side effects and cumulative pethidine compared to PCA. Therefore, this system is as effective as PCA in providing pain relief after surgical intervention.

Junior Anesthesiologist-Based Consultant-Supervised APS [52]

This is widely used in the United Kingdom and Australia. The APS is staffed each weekday by one of a pool of interested anesthesiologists and one full-time registered nurse; 24 h cover is provided with a staff anesthesiologist on call.

Usually, the surgeon writes "acute pain service" below the patient's name on the operating lists, but also the operating room anesthesiologist or any member of the nursing staff may refer a patient to the APS after discussion with the person responsible for APS. Preoperative patient education is mainly carried out by ward nursing staff accredited by APS. APS usually first comes into contact with the patient in the recovery room, and each patient is seen at least once each day and as often as necessary throughout the day. The analgesic technique started by the APS is continued until the patient is allowed free fluids or a light diet, when the oral or subcutaneous administration of a weak opioid or a non-steroidal anti-inflammatory drug can be commenced. Fourth-year medical students accompany anesthesiologists from the APS on routine ward rounds and, usually, complete for one semester a research project that is related to acute pain.

Nurse and Resident Anesthesiologist-Based Anesthesiologists on Duty Supervised APS

Our APS model at Cattinara Hospital in Trieste, Italy is a variation of the nurse-based model by Rawal [6], who has been our point of reference in the development of this model. The common goals of good APS are the following: to enrol every patient, to apply and advance new analgesic methods, to carry out clinical research in the area of postoperative pain management, to provide 24-h coverage, to use protocols, guidelines, and standard orders, to organize periodically educational programs and pain representative meetings, and to inform the patient about techniques for pain relief.

The end-point of APS might be to provide pain relief to patients. The literature indicates that the introduction of APS significantly improves in-patient perception of pain relief and patient satisfaction. According to a study published by de Leon Casasola et al. [53], there is also a reduction of up to 35% of hospital expenditure for patients receiving optimal analgesia.

The costs are quite different among the APS models according to the different drugs and techniques used. Moreover, it is very difficult to quantify the costs in medicine, because a lot of variables contribute and the total costs must be balanced with the benefits. The least-expensive among the proposed models is that of Murphy et al. [51], because the extra cost for personnel and devices is nothing. Ready's model, according to Rawal, is the most-expensive model. Its cost is about US$ 200-300 for the patient, because it includes several personnel such as staff anesthesiologist, resident anesthesiologist or pain fellow, pain nurse, pharmacist, physiotherapist, and sometimes psychologist, and consequently it appears unrealistic for most institutions.

The Rawal model is not expensive, because it requires few extra personnel, only the acute pain nurse. Its cost is about US$ 2-3 for the patient. But this cost is the result of a division between annual nurse salary, i.e., a fixed cost, and the number of patients treated within 1 year, i.e., a variable number. The annual salary of two nurses in Sweden is US$ 60.000 and the number of patients treated for 1 year at Orebro Hospital is about 20,000. The cost is hence US$ 2-3 for each patient. But this cost is strictly dependent on the number of patients treated per year. Moreover, it is independent of the cost of necessary devices to manage postoperative analgesia. For example, if the salary of two nurses is about US$ 35,000 and the number of APS-managed patients is about 650 for year, the costs would be about US$ 50 for each patient. Furthermore, the costs of the analgesic techniques have to be considered. In our APS, for example, there is a strong use of elastomeric pumps with a not negligible further cost. The cost is US$ 35 for 2 and 5 ml per hour pump, and more than US$ 50 for 0.5 ml per hour pump. The use of simple, effective, and inexpensive analgesic techniques should be encouraged.

A New Acute Pain Service Model

Nurse and Resident Anesthesiologist-Based Anesthesiologist on Duty Supervised APS

Since September 1998 we have started a nurse and resident anesthesiologist-based anesthesiologist-supervised APS. This service provides postoperative pain management for general, orthopedic, urological, vascular, plastic, thoracic, earnose-throat, and neurosurgical patients after acute and elective interventions.

The operating room anesthesiologist, at the end of surgery, fills in either the APS or standard postoperative paper. He is the first person responsible for the patient perioperative care and he decides, depending on the kind and length of surgery and the preoperative physical status of the patient, whether the patient enters the APS program. Generally, ASA (American Society of Anesthesiologists) ≤ 2 patients or those undergoing mild or short surgery return to the surgical wards directly with analgesic and monitoring orders written by the staff anesthesiologist; the

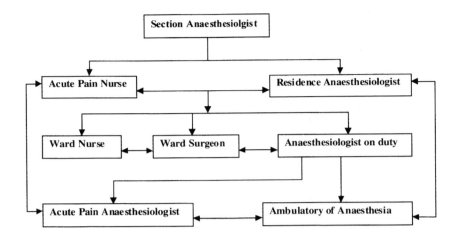

Fig. 1. Acute postoperative pain service organization at Cattinara Hospital, Trieste, Italy

monitoring routine and pain management on the ward is managed by the ward nurse and surgeon. On the other hand, ASA ≥ 2 patients or those undergoing major or long-duration surgery are followed directly by APS as summarized in Figure 1 and Table 1.

Every APS patient, either in the intensive care unit (ICU) or in a surgical ward, is asked to grade his or her pain severity by VAS every 3 h, and this intensity is recorded on the postoperative chart together with the other vital signs. Pain intensity is recorded more frequently (every hour) in ICU, in the first hours after surgery until VAS is ≥ 3, and in patients receiving PCA or epidural opioids. A specially

Table 1. Duties of health care members at Cattinara Hospital, Trieste, Italy

Health care member	Responsibility
Staff anesthesiologist	Responsible for perioperative care for his/her patients
Resident anesthesiologist and acute pain nurse	Daily rounds of all surgical wards. Liaison between surgeons and daily rounds of all surgical wards. Check VAS recording on charts. Solve technical problems (PCA, epidural, elastomeric pumps). Refer problem patients to staff anesthesiologist and anesthesiologist on duty
Acute pain anesthesiologist	Responsible for co-ordinating, supervising APS and educating hospital acute pain services

PCA, patient-controlled analgesia; *VAS*, visual analogic scales

trained acute pain nurse together with a resident anesthesiologist carry out a daily round of all surgery departments and record on the postoperative chart VAS, respiratory rate, heart rate, mean arterial pressure, diuresis, motor blockade, grade of sedation, nausea and vomiting, and other side effects. Whenever patients suffer pain, the acute pain anesthesiologist, during regular working hours, or the anesthesiologist on duty are asked to modify the pain management in order to maintain VAS below 3 or to avoid side effects due to the analgesic technique.

Audits are very important to measure and quantify the quality of pain management. Thus, utilizing a standardized questionnaire written as a five-grade survey developed by the American Pain Society, we collected data from 1,172 patient-respondents undergoing surgery. The satisfaction level of patients on pain service protocol was very high (Fig. 2) and the majority, if they ever needed surgery again, would like their pain treated in the same way (96.7%).

In summary, APS models are an important tool for improving postoperative pain management and consequently reducing morbidity, obtaining early alimentation, and rehabilitation. The key-points for improving acute pain management are the option for safety and simplicity of analgesic methods in order to accommodate increasing demands of quality assurance in pain and patient satisfaction, the regular measurement and recording of pain at the patient's beside, evidence-based decision making, the appropriate choice of drugs, the route, and mode of delivery, and the interdisciplinary approach to the postsurgical patient.

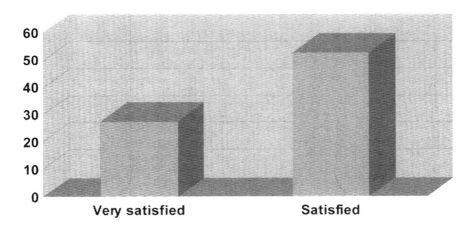

Fig. 2. Patient satisfaction level by analgesic modality

References

1. Maier C, Raetzel M, Wulf H (1994) Audit in 1989 and 1994 of the Department of Anaesthesiology and Intensive Care, Hospital of Christian-Albrechts-University, Schwanenweg 21, D 24105, Kiel, Germany
2. Neugebauer E, Hempel K, Sauerland S et al (1998) The status of perioperative pain therapy in Germany. Results of a representative, anonymous survey of 1000 surgical clinics. Chirurg 69:461-466
3. Donovan M, Dillon P, McGuire L (1983) Incidence and characteristics of pain in a sample of medical-surgical inpatients. Pain 30:69-78
4. Kuhn S, Cooke K, Collins M et al (1990) Perceptions of pain relief after surgery. BMJ 300:1687-1690
5. Owen H, McMillan V, Rogowski D (1990) Postoperative pain therapy: a survey of patients' expectations and their experiences. Pain 41:303-307
6. Rawal N (1994) Organization of acute pain services. Pain 57:117-123
7. Smith G (1991) Pain after surgery. Br J Anaesth 67:232-233
8. Rawal N (1996) Organization of postoperative pain service. In: Gullo A (ed) Anaesthesia, pain intensive care and emergency medicine. Springer-Verlag, Milan, Italy, pp 835-840
9. Watson A, Allen PR (1994) Influence of thoracic epidural analgesia on outcome after resection for esophageal cancer. Surgery 115:421-432
10. Yeager MP, Glass DD, Neff RK, Brinck-Johnsen T (1987) Epidural anesthesia and analgesia in high-risk surgical patients. Anesthesiology 66:729-736
11. Rawal N (1999) Organization of acute pain services. In: Gullo A (ed) Regional anaesthesia, analgesia and pain management. Springer-Verlag, Milan, Italy, pp 227-234
12. Shulman MS, Brebner J, Sandler A (1983) The effect of epidural morphine on postoperative pain relief and pulmonary function on thoracotomy patients. Anesthesiology 59:A192
13. Carli F (1999) Fast-track program for abdominal surgery. In: Gullo A (ed) Anaesthesia, pain intensive care and emergency. Springer, Milan, pp 211-218
14. Sharrock NE (1999) Fast-track anaesthesia and postoperative care: orthopaedic surgery In: Gullo A (ed) Anaesthesia, pain intensive care and emergency. Springer, Milan, pp 219-223
15. Rawal N, Hylander J, Nydahl PA et al (1997) Survey of postoperative analgesia following ambulatory surgery. Acta Anaesthesiol Scand 41:1017-1022
16. Kehlet H (1991) The surgical stress response: should it be prevented? Can J Surg 34:565-567
17. Kehlet H (1989) Surgical stress: the role of pain and analgesia. Br J Anaesth 63:189-195
18. Biebuyck J (1995) Epidural anesthesia and analgesia. Anesthesiology 82:1474-1506
19. Coderre TJ, Katz J, Vaccarino AL, Melzack R (1993) Contribution of central neuroplasticity to pathological pain: review of clinical and experimental evidence. Pain 52:259-285
20. Liu H, Mantyh PW, Basbaum AI (1997) NMDA-receptor regulation of substance P release from primary afferent nociceptors. Nature 386:721-724
21. Harris JA, Corsi M, Quartaroli M et al (1996) Upregulation of spinal glutamate receptors in chronic pain. Neuroscience 74:7-12
22. Schaible H-G, Jarrott B, Hope PJ, Duggan AW (1990) Release of immunoreactive substance P in the spinal cord during development of acute arthritis in the knee joint of the cat: a study with antibody microprobes. Brain Res 529:214-223
23. Curran T, Margan JI (1994) Fos: an immediate-early transcription factor in neurons. J Neur o-biol 26:403-412
24. Dickenson AH, Sullivan AF (1993) Combination therapy in analgesia: seeking synergy. Curr Opin Anesthesiol 6:861-865

25. Ready LB (1990) Acute postoperative pain. In: Miller RD (ed) Anesthesia, 3rd edn. Churchill Livingstone, New-York, pp 2135-2146
26. Dierking GW, Ostergaard E, Ostergard HT, Dahl JB (1994) The effects of wound infiltration with bupivacaine versus saline on postoperative pain and opioid requirements after herniorrhaphy. Acta Anaesthesiol Scand 38:289-292
27. Erichsen CJ, Vibits H, Dahl JB, Kehlet H (1995) Wound infiltration with ropivacaine and bupivacaine for pain after inguinal herniotomy. Acta Anaesthesiol Scand 39:67-70
28. Tverskoj M, Cozacov C, Ayache M et al (1990) Postoperative pain after inguinal herniorrhaphy with different types of anesthesia. Anesth Analg 70:29-35
29. Woolf CJ (1984) Long-term alterations in the excitability of the flexion relex produced by peripheral tissue injury in the chronic decerebrate rat. Pain 18:325-343
30. Jensen TS, Krebs B, Nielsen J, Rasmussen P (1985) Immediate and long-term phantom pain in amputees: incidence, clinical characteristics and relationship to pre-amputation pain. Pain 21:268-278
31. Page GG, McDonald JS, Ben-Eliyahu S (1998) Pre-operative versus postoperative administration of morphine: impact on the neuroendocrine, behavioural, and metastaticenhancing effects of surgery. Br J Anaesth 81:216-223
32. Gottschalk A, Smith DS, Jobes DR et al (1998) Pre-emptive epidural analgesia and recovery from radical prostatectomy. JAMA 279:1076-1082
33. Dahl JB, Daugaard JJ, Rasmussen B et al (1994) Immediate and prolonged effects of pre- versus postoperative epidural analgesia with bupivacaine and morphine on pain at rest and during mobilization after total knee arthroplasty. Acta Anaesthesiol Scand 38:557-561
34. Kundra P, Gurnani A, Bhattacharya A (1997) Preemptive epidural morphine for postoperative pain relief after lumbar laminectomy. Anesth Analg 85:135-138
35. Blake DW (1995) The general versus regional anaesthesia debate: time to re-examine the goals. Aust N Z J Surg 65:51-56
36. American Society of Anesthesiologists Task Force on Pain Management, Acute Pain Section (1995) A practical guidelines for acute pain management in the peri-operative setting. Anesthesiology 82:1071-1081
37. Max MB, Donovan M, Portenoy RK (1991) American Pain Society Quality Assurance Stan-dards for Relief of Acute Pain and Cancer Pain, Committee on Quality Assurance Standards, American Pain Society, In: Bond MR, Charlton JE, Woolf GJ (eds) Proceedings of the VIth World Congress on Pain. Elsevier, NewYork, pp 185-189
38. Ready LB, Edwards WT (1992) Management of acute pain. A practical guide. Task Force on Acute Pain. International Association for the Study of Pain. Seattle, IASP
39. Maier C, Kibbel K, Mercker S, Wulf H (1994) Postoperative pain therapy at general nursing stations. An analysis of eight years of experience at an anaesthesiological acute pain service. Anaesthesist 43:385-397
40. Ready BL, Oden R, Chadwick HS et al (1988) Development of an anesthesiology-based post-operative pain management service. Anesthesiology 68:100-106
41. Burstal R, Wegener F, Hayes C, Lantry G (1988) Epidural analgesia: prospective audit of 1062 patients. Anaesth Intensive Care 26:165-172
42. The Royal College of Surgeons of England and The College of Anaesthetists (1990) Commission on the provision of surgical services. Report of the Working Party on Pain after surgery. London: HMSO
43. Windsor AM, Glynn CJ, Mason DG (1996) National provision of acute pain services. Anaesthesia 51:228-231
44. Stacey BR, Rudy TE, Nelhaus D (1997) Management of patient-controlled analgesia: a comparison of primary surgeons and dedicated pain service. Anesth Analg 85:130-134
45. Saidman LJ (1988) The anesthesiologist outside the operating room: a new and exciting opportunity. Anesthesiology 68:100-106

46. Sartain JB, Barry JJ (1999) The impact of an acute pain service on postoperative pain management. Anaesth Intensive Care 27:375-380
47. Macintyre PE, Runciman WB, Webb R (1990) An acute pain service in an Australian teaching hospital: the first year. Med J Aust 153:417-421
48. A Report by the American Society of Anesthesiologists Task Force on Pain Management, Acute Pain Section (1995) Practice guidelines for acute pain management in the perioperative setting. Anesthesiology 82:1071-1081
49. Miaskowski C, Crews J, Ready LB et al (1999) Anesthesia-based services improve the quality of postoperative pain management. Pain 80:23-29
50. Zimmermann LD, Stewart J (1993) Postoperative pain management and acute pain service activity in Canada. Can J Anaesth 40:568-575
51. Murphy DF, Graziotti P, Chalkiadis G, McKenna M (1994) Patient-controlled analgesia: a comparison with nurse-controlled intravenous opioid infusions. Anaesth Intensive Care 22; 5:589-592
52. Macintyre PE, Runciman WB, Webb RK (1990) An acute pain service in an Australian teaching hospital: the first year. Med J Aust 153:417-421
53. de Leon Casasola OA, Parker BM, Lema MJ et al (1994) Epidural analgesia versus intravenous patient-controlled analgesia. Differences in the post-operative course of cancer patients. Reg Anesth 19:307-315
54. Rawal N (1997) Organization of acute pain services – a low-cost model. Acta Anaesthesiol Scand [Suppl]111:188-190
55. Rawal N (1995) Acute pain services in Europe: A 17-nation survey. Reg Anesth 20:S85

Chapter 11

Postoperative Functional Pain Management

F. NICOSIA

Despite all the improvements in anaesthesia and surgery, patients still have problems after the operations. Many of them have injured, induced organ dysfunction (surgical stress syndrome). All patients have pain and many experience nausea and vomiting, which may limit oral feeding; fatigue and inability to work are very common. A few patients suffer major postoperative complications al though the operation was technically successful. Pulmonary, thrombo-embolic and cardiac complications are among the most common life-threatening consequences of surgery.

There are data [1] that demonstrate Regional Anaesthesia (RA) + fast track are good for the patients. Fast recovery is supposed to be the aim of modern health institutions. In fact the rapid advances in anaesthesia and analgesia have made fast-track surgery possible. Local and RA can shorten recovery room time and help mobilize patients earlier by protecting them from surgical stress and postoperative pain during recovery from minor and major surgery.

Examples From the Literature

- **Fast track for carotid endarterectomy**
- Preoperative education
- Local anaesthesia
- Stress-free surgery
- Hospital stay 1.3 days (84%, 1 day)

- **Fast track for mastectomy** [2, 3]
- Preoperative education
- Drainage
- Ambulatory
- No increased risk
- Improved arm mobilization
- A total of 256 mastectomies
- Paravertebral block with local anaesthetics (96%, 24 h hospital stay)

- **Fast track for herniectomy** [4]
- Preoperative education
- Infiltration local anaesthesia

- No preoperative tests
- Walk in-walk out regimen
- Postoperative NSAIDs

- **Fast track for pulmonary lobectomy** [5]
- Fifty consecutive patients
- Selective use of intensive care (12%)
- Hospital stay = 3 days

- **Fast track for colonic surgery** [6]
- Patient information
- Thoracic epidural analgesia
- No drain
- Transverse incision
- Early mobilization
- Cisaspride and magnesium
- Two-day hospital stay whatever the preoperative conditions
    1. Day of surgery: out of bed for 3 h, drink proteins
    2. Day 1: 8 h out of bed, no i.v. line, remove urinary catheter, plan discharge
    3. Day 2: normal activity

Every day the nurses have to fill out of the patient's chart. The nurse should justify why the patient is unable to do the programme.

- **Fast track for radical prostatectomy** [7]
- Preoperative education
- Epidural
- NSAIDs + acetaminophen
- No use of drains
- A total of 180 patients
- Hospital stay, 1.3 days

Why shouldn't all operations be event-less? The pathophysiological background is perhaps the most important subject of research in the field of surgical interventions. The key issue is to have every operation pain and risk free. The purpose is to accelerate patient recovery and reduce postoperative morbidity so as to enable the patients to be active and thus reduce hospital stay. As a consequence, costs will be reduced as well.

According to Khelet [8] many factors are involved in perioperative care and may limit recovery:
- Pain
- Nausea and vomiting
- Hypoxaemia
- Sleep disturbances
- Cardiac morbidity
- Immobilization

- Semi starvation
- Fatigue
- Conventions

Patient Recovery

Postsurgical recovery should be evaluated in terms of both speed and quality and can be divided into three main phases: early, intermediate and late.

The assessment of early phase recovery involves the measurement of physiological parameters such as alertness, respiration and cardiocirculatory activity. Intermediate recovery can last until the patient is considered able to reach "home readiness" and to rest at home under the care of a responsible adult. Street fitness is the late condition when the patient is able to return to normal activity and work.

The time spent for intermediate and late recovery may be influenced by both drugs and techniques used by the anaesthetists. It should be, for instance, emphasized that rapid postoperative wake up may not correlate with a patient's rapid return to normal function [1].

Postoperative events can be improved by using prevention and care. RA has been demonstrated to be extremely useful for this purpose. It is well recognized that the surgical event is an injury and all techniques for patientprotection should be adopted. Keeping the temperature normal in the patients and giving good anaesthesia and good postoperative analgesia are extremely important. Surgeons and anaesthesiologists have to understand that RA is the most important anaesthetic method for patient protection. During standard general anaesthesia the afferent input may still reach the spinal cord, producing reflexes in the endocrine and metabolic system. The autonomic response to several organs will inhibit pulmonary function, increase cardiac demand and trigger what is known as stress-induced organ dysfunction. Unlike standard general anaesthesia, if epidural or spinal anaesthesia is used and continued into the postoperative period, we can block those responses and blunt the stress response, without inducing autonomic dysfunction etc. This also provides the most efficient pain relief when RA is continued through 48 to 72 h postoperatively.

A meta-analysis of all the Randomised Controlled Trials (RCT) comparing general and RA has considered about 10,000 patients. The risk of intraoperative bleeding is decreased; the need for postoperative transfusion is also decreased and so are all major complications – thrombosis, myocardial infarction, and even mortality within 30 days was highly reduced (Finucane, personal communication).

Ileus

Postoperatively, ileus is something surgeons believe to be unavoidable, perhaps even necessary, a reflex response. In fact, we have the afferent from the surgical wound to the spinal cord and the afferent to the bowel which inhibits motility. If epidural blockade is used, we can block the reflex. There have been studies comparing epidural bupivacaine and epidural opiates or systemic opiates on postoperative intestinal function. Several studies have shown a difference in gastrointestinal discharge, anticipated for about 2 days [9-11]. That means that the patient can be fed earlier if continuous epidural local anaesthetic is administered after abdominal operations.

Oxygen saturation

Postoperative hypoxaemia is well known. After major abdominal interventions, oxygen saturation decreases and recovers after days. During the night, there are also episodic desaturations and at that time we can increase the heart rate. That means that during the night there is less substrate for the heart and more work. The supply-demand ratio is negative. That way postoperative hypoxaemia may contribute to cardiac complications, not to mention wound complications, cerebral dysfunction, confusion, delirium, and hallucinations. Therefore postoperative oxygenation should improve. This can be done by simply mobilizing the patients. If the patient is mobilized hypoxaemia does not appear.

There is an effect of perioperative oxygen on surgical wound infection. A randomised study on 500 operated patients [12] showed less wound infections (from 11% to 6%) just providing good oxygen saturation.

Therefore, oxygen and the mechanisms of hypoxaemia to be treated are very important for improving outcome. The simplest method of improving oxygenation is mobilizing the patients. The issue is: how can we mobilize patients in pain in the immediate postoperative period? We can give analgesics, namely small dosages of opiates and local anaesthetics, avoiding systemic opiates insofar as possible.

Immobilization

Immobilization is the most important factor for postoperative morbidity, since it stimulates catabolism, which in turn is responsible for loss of muscle mass and function. As a consequence, fatigue and inability to work are the common symptoms of operated patients.

There are three major ways of reducing fatigue, loss of muscle mass and function:
- Reduce catabolic response by using epidurals
- Prevent immobilization by optimal pain-relieving techniques
- Avoid semi-starvation

Effect of postoperative immobilization
- Catabolism   ⇑
- Pulmonary function   ⇓
- O$_2$ saturation   ⇓
- Muscle function   ⇓
- Orthostatic reflexes ⇓
- Fluid excretion   ⇓

Standards

The problem of the postoperative period cannot be solved by a single mode of treatment because it is a multifactorial problem [8]. Therefore, the technique to improve outcome needs to be multimodal. In the postoperative period surgeons have numerous conventional methods. For instance, there are more than 30 CRT controlled randomized trials which show that we should not use naso-gastric tube routinely. This also applies to unnecessary drains: there are meta-analyses indicating that drains should not be used routinely [13]. In fact they may hinder rehabilitation. The essence for the control of perioperative pathophysiology is diagrammatically shown here below.

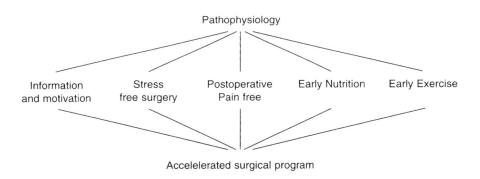

How can postoperative morbidity be avoided?

Anaesthetists and surgeons are faced with many important factors correlated to postoperative morbidity. Preoperative risk factors are usually considered very important. However, they are so important because the postoperative period is so bad. If we transform surgery to mini-invasive surgery, if we transform anaesthesia to "patient protection" in addition to "surgery facilitation", and if we rethink postoperative care, then fast track surgical procedures are possible because they prevent organ functions from decreasing.

As anaesthesiologists we must focus on anaesthetic intraoperative management and postoperative care.

The use of RA is, paradoxically, more important for the outcome of major surgery than of minor surgery, since the former causes more organ dysfunction than the latter. Therefore, in major surgery there is a greater need for intraoperative protection and postoperative multimodal support than in minor operations, independently of the subjective pain sensation.

References

1. Rudkin GE (1997) Patient recovery and discharge. In: Millar JM, Rudkin GE, Hitchcock M (eds) Practical anaesthesia and analgesia for day surgery. Bios Scientific, pp 218-222
2. Coveney E, Weltz CR, Greengrass R et al (1998) Use of paravertebral block anaesthesia in the surgical treatment of breast cancer. Ann Surg 222:496-501
3. Bonnema J, Van Wresch AM, van Geel AN et al (1998) Medical and psychosocial effects of early discharge after surgery for breast cancer: randomised trial. BMJ 316:1267-1271
4. Callensen T, Beck K, Kehlet H et al (1998) The feasibility, safety and cost of infiltration anaesthesia fir hernia repair. Anaesthesia 53:31-35
5. Tovar EA, Roethe RA, Weissig MD et al (1998) One day admission for lung lobectomy: an initial result of a clinical pathway. Ann Thorac Surg 65:803-806
6. Kehlet H, Mogensen T (1999) Two days hospital stay after open sigmoidectomy. Br J Surg 86:227-230
7. Worwag E, Chodak GW (1998) Overnight hospitalisation after radical prostatectomy. Anesth Analg 87:62-67
8. Kehlet H (1997) Multimodal approach to control postoperative pathophysiology and rehabilitation. Br J Anaesth 78:606-617
9. Carpenter R (1996) Gastrointestinal benefits of regional anesthesia/analgesia. Reg Anesth 21 [Suppl 6]:13-17
10. Thorn SE, Watturl M, Kallander A et al (1994) Effect of epidural morphine and epidural bupivacaine on gastrointestinal motility during the fasted state and after food intake. Acta Anaesthsiol Scand 38:57-62
11. Crawford ME, Moiniche S, Orback J et al (1996) Orthostatic hypotention during postoperative continuous thoracic epidural bupivacaine-morphine in patients undergoing abdominal surgery. Anesth Analg 83:1028-1032
12. Greif R, Akca O, Horn EP et al (2000) Supplemental perioperative oxygen to reduce the incidence of surgical wound infection. New Engl J Med 342:161-167
13. Benoist S, Panis Y, Denet C et al (1999) Optimal duration of urinary drainage after rectal resection: A randomised controlled trial. Surgery 125:135-141

Chapter 12

Timing for Narcotic Drugs in Terminal Illness

S. MERCADANTE

Pain is a major symptom in cancer. About 30% of patients undergoing oncological treatment and 70% of patients with advanced disease suffer pain due to different causes, such as tumor progression or treatment-related syndromes.

Cancer pain is less than optimally controlled all over the world. Physicians' knowledge and attitudes to pain management are likely to contribute to undertreatment [1]. Although cancer pain is still undertreated, instruments exist for controlling this feared symptom of advanced cancer. The availability of guidelines and accumulating clinical experience have greatly improved the possibility of satisfactory pain control for most patients with advanced cancer [2]. Current treatment is based on the World Health Organization's concept of an analgesic ladder which involves a simple stepwise approach to the use of analgesic drugs. However, it is essentially a framework of principles rather than a rigid protocol. Different alternative procedures may increase the possibilities of pain control and personalization of therapy is strongly encouraged. What is imperative is the pain control at any stage of disease. Pain is experienced by one-third to one-half of those who are ambulatory or are receiving active antineoplastic therapy and more than two-thirds of those with advanced disease. Pain has been found to be prevalent among well-functioning ambulatory patients and substantially compromises function in approximately half of the patients who experience it [3]. Chronic pain must be treated as it can interact significantly with many facets of daily living. Therefore, factors that govern the decision about the appropriate selection of pharmaceutical agent include the severity of pain, and not the stage of the illness.

Symptomatic drug treatment is used in an integrated way with disease-modifying therapy and non-drug measures. Drug therapy is the cornerstone of cancer pain management. It is effective, relatively low risk, inexpensive, and usually works quickly. An essential principle in using medications to manage cancer pain is to individualize the regimen to the patient [4].

Non opioid analgesics are effective for relief of mild pain, and have an opioid-sparing effect that helps reduce adverse effects when given with opioids for moderated to severe pain. Although non opioid analgesics are used first in the hierarchy of the WHO three step ladder recommendation, opioids should not be withheld when these drugs are no longer effective. Indeed, higher doses of non opioid analgesics produce serious adverse effects with prolonged used and an appropriate switch to opioids is strongly recommended, regardless of the status of the illness. Once a primary therapy has been able to control the causes of pain, opioid doses can be gradually reduced without producing serious consequences and eventually stopped.

Causes of Escalating Opioid Doses

The fear to increase the opioid dose is the most important limiting factor in the management of cancer pain at any time of the disease. The need for escalating doses is a complex phenomenon and may have numerous explanations. If pain is due to progressive disease, tolerance cannot be inferred to exist. If dose escalation is needed in the absence of other obvious causes, tolerance may be the explanation, but the term tolerance itself is used to describe multiple processes.

So-called associative tolerance is related to conditioning and so-called pharmacological tolerance is related to the pharmacology of the drug. Pharmacological tolerance may be dispositional, due to pharmacokinetic changes, or, more commonly, pharmacodynamic, due to a decline in analgesic effects related to some process of neural adaptation.

These processes are characterized by large intraindividual and interindividual variability. Tolerance to different opioid effects develops at varying rates and can occur quickly after acute dosing or accrue more gradually with repeated dosing [5, 6]. The development of tolerance to adverse effects is usually favourable, enlarging the therapeutic window, whereas analgesic tolerance is a process that reduces opioid responsiveness.

The development of tolerance can be constant over the course of long-term administration or can appear to have an accelerated phase at beginning of the treatment. The repeated administration of opioids can lead to the development of tolerance, which is an important element in the concept of opioid responsiveness. In one survey, relatively high opioid doses and the need for a rapid increase in opioid dose predicted a poor outcome in pain relief [7]. This does not mean that tolerance is the cause of using such high doses of opioids.

The assessment of potential analgesic tolerance in cancer patients is constrained by the complexity of the clinical situation. Increasing activity in nociceptive pathways, which may be due to mechanical factors, biochemical changes related to the progression of a lesion or to the development of either peripheral or central neuropathic processes, in which case the term tolerance does not apply, may explain declining analgesic effects during opioid treatment in cancer patients.

It is possible, however, that some patients with longstanding pain or neuropathic pain, who develop the need for escalating doses do so because of mechanisms related to pharmacodynamic tolerance. Too little is known about the mechanisms of these conditions to state with certainty that poor opioid responsiveness due to neuropathic pain is not related to tolerance, at least in some cases.

The reduced antinociceptive effects of morphine associated with hyperalgesia in animal models of neuropathic pain, which develop in the absence of daily exposure to morphine [8], may be similar to the clinical situation and could also involve tolerance.

Tumor on its own may be responsible for a poor response to morphine. For example, impaired opioid responsiveness has been reported in an infant with localized metastasis to the midbrain periaqueductal gray, presumably due to loss of tissue with opioid-specific cell bodies [9].

Thus, the clinical picture may be complicated by the progressive course of the illness or related events that require increasing doses. Patients who are given opioids for chronic pain and are clinically stable usually remain on a stable dosage for long period after achieving adequate analgesia. Several studies have indicated that increases in morphine doses during a chronic morphine treatment were related to punctual events, such as surgery, invasive exploration, or a progression of disease, generating an increase in pain, supporting the view that development of tolerance to opioids is unlikely to be the driving force for loss of analgesia in patients who have alternative reasons for increasing pain. There appears to be general acceptance that the most common reason for escalating opioid doses is the progress of the underlying malignant disease, which causes increasing pain [8, 10]. However, the progression of disease often occurs with little or no pain, as in the development of pulmonary or hepatic metastases and the opioid escalation can become unexpectedly rapid without evident progression of disease or modifications on the type of pain.

Opioid doses often can be decreased if pain is relieved by another treatment [11, 12]. This observation further suggests that the mechanism of dose escalation may not involve tolerance when the underlying disease is active or progressing. This reduction of opioid dosage and the rapid return of opioid sensitivity that this implies cannot be explained if the gradual process of neural adaptation consistent with pharmacodynamic tolerance is the major factor [13].

Patients receiving high dose treatment with opioids can experience respiratory depression following total pain relief obtained by other methods. The occurrence of severe opioid-induced side effects following interventions such as a nerve block suggests that mechanisms other than tolerance may also be involved when non analgesic effects decline or fail to appear during opioid administration. Therefore, tolerance to non analgesic effects presumably occurs, but other factors also may allow the patient to tolerate higher doses of opioids. Again, phenomenon of changing dose-response relationship is not uniform in clinical practice and caution should be observed when extrapolating experimental data.

From the clinical perspective, this analysis suggests that analgesic tolerance rarely represents a limiting factor during opioid treatment. In cancer pain, there is no maximum dose to define opioid unresponsiveness. That is the dose-response for analgesia shows no ceiling effect. Although the dose-response may shift to the right during treatment, dose escalation may still provide analgesia unless important side effects occur.

If opioid doses are gradually increased, very high dosages are generally well tolerated and not associated with the risk of the most feared side effect, respiratory depression. Indeed, the presence of pain stimulates respiration and attenuates morphine-induced respiratory depression in an intensity-dependent fashion [14]. Although it is often observed that tolerance to respiratory depression rapidly develops with chronic treatment [15], persistent pain itself may be part of the mechanism that allows dose escalation.

Although tolerance to analgesic or non-analgesic effects may be a relevant factor, it is ultimately the balance between pain relief and toxicity that defines responsiveness. A propensity to side effects, which may be related to advanced age or any of numerous conditions frequently observed in advanced cancer patients, including organ failure and concomitant drug administration, may be the most important consideration in many cases [16].

Opioid tolerance and physical dependence do not equate with addiction. The predictable consequences of long-term opioid administration, tolerance and dependence, are often confused with psychological dependence (addiction), that manifests as drug abuse. This misunderstanding can lead to ineffective prescribing, administering, or dispensing of opioids for cancer pain. The result is undertreatment. Clinicians may be reluctant to give high doses of opioids to patients with cancer pain because of a fear of serious adverse effects. The clinician's ethical duty to benefit the patient by relieving pain supports increasing doses, even at risk of side effects. Because many patients with cancer pain become tolerant to most adverse effects during long-term opioid therapy, the clinician's fear of shortening life by increasing opioid doses is usually unfounded.

Opioid Tolerance in Clinical Setting

Morphine is the standard step 3 opioid analgesic against which others are measured and is the most widely available in a variety of oral formulations. Generally, the oral route is preferred because of ease of administration, and it is usually cost-effective. The appropriate dose is the amount that controls pain with the fewest adverse effects. The need for increased doses of opioid often reflects progression of disease [2]. When patients cannot take oral medications, other less invasive routes, such as subcutaneous and transdermal ones, should be offered.

In some circumstances, however, dose escalation may be due to opioid analgesic tolerance rather than progressive disease. The variability in analgesic or adverse effect response to different opioid analgesics is relatively common and is probably due to an incomplete cross-tolerance among opioids. This phenomenon is frequently attributed to differential opioid receptor affinities. Tolerance develops independently at each receptor subtype in response to the binding of a drug and its intrinsic activity. Changes in the receptor-effector relationship may also occur over the course of the illness with prolonged morphine exposure. It has also been suggested that the phenomenon depends on genetic factors. As a result, individual receptor profile and specific clinical conditions may influence the final effects in terms of analgesia or side effects.

The phenomenon of asymmetric cross-tolerance could also be due to differences in agonist efficacies, rather than receptor selectivities. According to the theory of receptor occupancy, different opioids may produce equivalent pain relief while occupying different proportions of the available receptors. Morphine tends to occupy more receptors to give an effect, producing a greater tolerance effect, due to high occupancy requirements, than high-efficacy agonists, such as sufentanil, which has a higher receptor reserve. Dose-response changes with progressive increases in stimulus intensity have been demonstrated. With an increase in stimulus intensity, sufentanil showed a smaller shift in its dose response curve than morphine, which showed a greater reduction in the maximum effect and increased occupancy requirements. This observation supports the receptor occupancy theory. Several opioids, including methadone, fentanyl and sufentanil have been demonstrated to have a much higher efficacy than morphine, due to a higher receptor reserve than morphine [17].

These experimental data may explain the loss of efficacy with increasing doses of morphine. A switching to an alternative opioid with a higher efficacy may reverse the reduced response to morphine.

On the other hand patients' analgesic response may depend on their morphine: metabolite ratio. While morphine-6-glucuronide (M6G) is an active metabolite of morphine that has analgesic properties, morphine-3-glucuronide (M3G), the major metabolite of morphine, has a negligible affinity for opioid receptors and is considered to be devoid of analgesic activity. On the contrary, experimental studies have shown that M3G produces neuroexcitatory and antianalgesic effects, so mimicking tolerance to analgesic effects of morphine, and adverse effects with increasing doses or prolonged administration [18].

The asymmetry observed in the development of tolerance could also be due to changes in pharmacokinetics, including adsorption, distribution, metabolism, and specific disease.

These preclinical data are also demonstrated by the reduction in the equianalgesic dose when switching opioids, due to possible incomplete cross tolerance. With high dosages, there is a risk of metabolite accumulation and the occurrence of relevant adverse effects. Thus, the possibility of rapid development of tolerance to the analgesia effects of opioids may be a problem in these circumstances. There is no clear indication of what causes tolerance and what percentage of patients could be expected to develop tolerance in a presumed absence of disease progression.

Assessing the patient's response to several different oral opioids is usually advisable before abandoning the previous approach in favour of more complex invasive techniques. Switching from one opioid to another one may improve the balance between analgesia and adverse effects in a large number of cases, avoiding recurrence to such complicated approaches, due to a different profile in inducing tolerance among different opioids in individuals.

In conclusion, opioids remain the cornerstone of the management of cancer pain. There is no doubt that these drugs should be indicated in the presence of high level of pain intensity, regardless of the stage of disease. The best opioid should be offered to individuals after assessing the response, before providing alternative complex approaches.

References

1. Cleeland CS, Gonin R, Hatfield AK et al (1994) Pain and its treatment in outpatients with metastatic cancer. N Engl J Med 330:592-596
2. Hanks GW, De Conno F, Ripamonti C et al (1996) Morphine in cancer pain: modes of administration. BMJ 312:823-826
3. Portenoy RK, Miransky J, Thaler H et al (1992) Pain in ambulatory patients with lung or colon cancer. Cancer 70:1616-1624
4. Mercadante S (1999) Treatment and outcome of cancer pain in advanced cancer patients followed at home. Cancer 85:1849-1858

5. Collin E, Cesselin F (1991) Neurobiological mechanisms of opioid tolerance and dependence. Clin Pharmacol 14:465-488
6. Portenoy RK (1995) Tolerance to opioid analgesics: clinical aspects. Cancer Surveys 21:49-65
7. Bruera E, MacMillan D, Hanson J, MacDonald RN (1989) The Edmonton staging system for cancer pain : preliminary report. Pain 37:203-210
8. Mao J, Price D, Mayer DJ (1985) Experimental mononeuropathy reduces the antinociceptive effects of morphine: implications for common intracellular mechanisms involved in morphine tolerance and neuropathic pain. Pain 61:353-364
9. Collins JJ, Berde CB, Grier HE et al (1995) Massive opioid resistance in an infant with a localized metastasis to the midbrain periaqueductal gray. Pain 1995:271-275
10. Collin E, Poulain P, Gauvain-Piquard A et al (1993) Is disease progression the major factor in morphine "tolerance" in cancer pain treatment? Pain 55:319-326
11. Portenoy RK, Foley KM (1986) Chronic use of opioid analgesics in non-malignant pain: report of 38 cases. Pain 25:171-186
12. Coyle N, Weaver S, Breibart W, Portenoy RK (1994) Delirium as a contributing factor to crescendo pain: three case reports, J Pain Symptom Manage 9:44-47
13. Galer BS, Coyle N, Pasternak GW, Portenoy RK (1992) Individual variability in the response to different opioids: report of five cases. Pain 49:87-91
14. Borgbjerg FM, Nielsen K, Franks J (1996) Experimental pain stimulates respiration and attenuates morphine-induced respiratory depression: a controlled study in human volunteers. Pain 64:123-128
15. Mercadante S, Portenoy RK (2000) Opioid poorly responsive cancer pain. Part 1. Clinical considerations. J Pain Symptom Manage, in press
16. Walsh TD (1984) Opiates and respiratory function in advanced cancer. Recent Results. Cancer Res 89:115-117
17. Mercadante S (1999) Opioid rotation in cancer pain: rationale and clinical aspects. Cancer 86:1856-1866
18. Mercadante S (1999) The role of morphine metabolites in cancer pain. Palliat Med 13:95-104

Chapter 13

Ethical Decisions in Terminal Illness

D. Kettler, M. Mohr

Ethical decisions in terminal illness involve conflicts such as whether to withhold or to withdraw treatment, to perform a resuscitative attempt, or to allocate limited and expensive resources. Decision making has been complicated by the rapid progress in technology in intensive care and emergency medicine. A terminally ill patient is frequently unable to communicate and to express his or her will and preferences. Physicians often become a surrogate decision maker and have the responsibility of deciding whether to limit or withhold futile care. However, in terminal illness the definition of futility is not clear and is still a matter of discussion. Therefore, in the intensive and palliative care setting consensus among the diverse group of health care professionals is especially relevant. Despite a wide variety of personal beliefs and cultural and religious differences, decisions in ethical conflicts should be based on generally accepted principles such as respect for autonomy, beneficence, nonmaleficence, and justice.

Ethical Deliberation: Principles and Rules

It might be argued that the nature of intensive care and emergency medicine, demanding immediate and often irreversible interventions, makes ethical deliberation impossible. However, clinical practice in terminal illness – just as that of any other medical procedure – must be guided by sound ethical reasoning. Beauchamp and Childress [1] defined four levels in the hierarchy of ethical justification (Fig. 1): ethical theories, principles, rules and particular judgments and actions.

Medical treatment, e.g. the initiation of ventilatory support, can be characterized as an action, which is the basic level of moral deliberation. The decision to start artificial ventilation is based on the medical judgment that a person is suffering from dyspnea and hypoxia. The decision to intubate and ventilate is justified by the moral rule – and now we are approaching the second level of moral justification – that the victim of respiratory distress has the right to survive and to receive respiratory support. In addition, the obligation to give aid also belongs to the generally accepted moral rules in medicine.

Moral rules are based on ethical principles, which constitute the third hierarchical level. Beauchamp and Childress [1] suggest four principles for acceptance as guidance for taking action in medicine:
- The principle of respect for autonomy

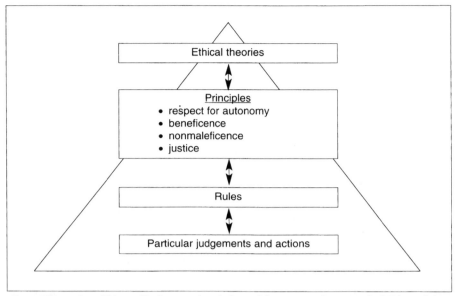

Fig. 1. Hierarchy of biomedical reasoning (adapted from Beauchamp and Childress [1])

- The principle of beneficence
- The principle of nonmaleficence
- The principle of justice

The precise distinction between rules and principles is controversial. Principles are characterized as more general and fundamental than moral rules, and serve to justify the rules. Rules – such as guidelines and consensus statements – are more related to a specific context and are more restricted in scope. Principles are conceived as binding, but not absolutely binding. This permits each principle to have weight without the determination of a ranking [1]. Which principle overrides in a case of conflict will depend on the context which – in particular in terminal illness – always has unique features.

Ethical theories – the top level in bioethical reasoning - are integrated bodies of principles and rules, depending on individual considerations about the world. Diverse scientific, metaphysical, and religious beliefs may underlie our interpretation of a situation and our personal ethical theory. Ethical theories may serve to justify the principles, the rules, and the particular judgment. But due to their abstractness, these theories are often far away from clinical practice. Discussing basic moral principles avoids discussing different types of ethical theories, such as utilitarian or deontological theories [1].

The principles are principles in the sense of being *principia*. The American philosopher Engelhardt pointed out that bioethical principles indicate foundations for major elements of moral life, the sources of particular areas of moral rights and obligations [2]. They constitute the beginnings, commencements, or origins of particular areas of moral life. They are principles in the sense of indicating the roots for the justification of moral concerns in health care [2].

The Principle of Respect for Autonomy

Physicians do not have the right to treat patients without their consent: *Voluntas aegroti suprema lex est*. The right to consent or to refuse a treatment is based on the principle of respect for autonomy. Physicians must obtain informed consent from patients, even in the terminally ill, before undertaking procedures. Five elements have been proposed as the components of informed consent [1]:
- Competence
- Disclosure of information
- Understanding of information
- Voluntariness
- Authorization

The process of informed consent from a competent patient involves adequate disclosure and understanding of information concerning the consequences of the intervention and the potential alternatives so that a voluntary decision to authorize or refuse a medical procedure can be made. In bioethical contexts, competence implies the ability to make a decision as to whether or not a therapeutic or diagnostic procedure should be undertaken. The patient's decision should reflect rational considerations based on information given by the physician.

The process of disclosure includes information on the nature of the disease, prognosis and risks and benefits of the various options. However, there seems to be a considerable lack of understanding among patients of medical procedures and their prognostic implications. Disclosure of information might change a patient's attitude. For example, it has been demonstrated that providing knowledge about cardiopulmonary resuscitation (CPR) and survival rates can lead to a marked decrease in consent to resuscitation in the elderly. Interviews performed in a geriatric practice revealed that a high percentage (41%) of outpatients would opt for CPR if they had a cardiac arrest during acute illness [3]. In case of cardiac arrest during a chronic or terminal illness (life expectancy less than 1 year) the number of patients choosing CPR decreased considerably (11%). There was a further reduction in acceptance of resuscitation attempts after additional information was disclosed as to the probable rate of survival for both conditions: then only 22% would still opt for CPR during an acute illness (arrest survival rate 10%–17%). Knowing the arrest survival probability of 0%–5% during a chronic or terminal disease, only 5% of the elderly patients would still choose to undergo CPR [3]. These results emphasize the essential need for prognostic information for the patient to make an informed decision concerning different treatment options.

Many approaches tend to distort informed consent by suggesting that disclosure is the key item in the act of giving informed consent. Informed consent should not be understood primarily in terms of the obligation to inform patients. Competence seems to be the threshold element in the process. Does the patient have the ability

to perform the task to authorize or to reject a treatment? Does he or she have the decision making capacity? The Task Force on Ethics of the Society of Critical Care Medicine [4] stated in the consensus report of 1990 that the capacity to decide includes the following abilities:
- To appreciate the significant characteristics of one's condition
- To appreciate the impact of the main treatment options
- To judge the relationship of options to one's beliefs and values
- To reason and to deliberate about one's choices
- To communicate decisions in a meaningful manner

In critical and palliative care medicine, due to the underlying disease process, the patient is often unable to communicate and to express his or her will and preferences. Particular in end-stage disease, many patients have lost consciousness and, thus, decision-making capacity. The patient is incapable of accepting or rejecting treatment. Thus, in many circumstances treatment decisions have to be made without a patient's involvement. Often, consent to treat is presumed. Nevertheless, physicians and all others involved have an obligation to serve as the patient's advocate by attempting to avoid undue harm. Such behavior might be judged as a paternalistic approach in medical practice. However, in the terminally ill patient this should be considered primarily as an attempt to do what is assumed to be in the patient's best interests. In some instances, the imminent need to treat makes it impossible to elucidate the patient's preferences first. When there is insufficient time to obtain consent from a patient or a patient's surrogate, physicians are under the general moral obligation to provide the kind of care a reasonable or prudent person would be likely to expect under the circumstances. The moral criterion becomes not actual consent but presumed consent [5].

Foregoing Treatment

Withholding and withdrawing life-support is one of the most important ethical issues in critical and palliative care medicine. In some ICUs approximately 50% of the deaths occur following withdrawal of therapy [5]. Today almost 90% of critical care professionals state that they are withholding or withdrawing life-prolonging treatment from patients they consider to have irreversible and terminal disease [5]. Both preservation of life and quality of life must be weighed when making decisions concerning withholding and withdrawing life-sustaining treatments [4]. Ethically, it is often stated that there is no difference between not initiating treatment and withdrawing it; a decision to withdraw a treatment already initiated should not necessarily be regarded as more problematic than a decision not to initiate a treatment [4].

Sometimes the start of life-saving or life-sustaining treatments might be necessary to permit full evaluation of the patient's condition and long-term prognosis, and later on, after all information is available and the development of the disease process is known, the decision of whether to withdraw these therapies might be required. Practically, the withdrawal or revision of treatment refers to the cessation of all therapeutic support when it is considered futile to continue treatment with the goal of curing the patient. In this context, it is often advanced life support that is withdrawn, but termination of treatment might include basic life support as well (e.g., hydration, nutrition). However, the removal of life support from a patient should not be regarded as an abandonment of the patient by the healthcare team [4]. Healthcare professionals have the obligation to continue supportive care and treatment for pain and suffering. To this end, analgesics and anxylitics may be used, even though they may, as a side-effect, depress cardiorespiratory function and indirectly hasten death [4].

Consensus among the members of the intensive care team (including the nursing staff) as well as between ICU physician and referring physicians is crucial. This must be obtained prior to discussion with the patient or relatives. Decision-making with families should not be rushed. Facilitators may be very helpful, and the health care team should work with the family towards making a unanimous decision regarding life support for incompetent patients. An institutional mechanism such as an ethics committee should be available. In addition, there might be an affirmative professional duty to refer the patient to other qualified practitioners. If these mechanisms fail, the courts may need to be involved. If a unanimous decision to withdraw therapy cannot be reached, treatment is usually continued [5]. Medical ethicists and patient advocates agree, in principle, that life-support measures can be discontinued when they are unwanted and futile; however, there is consistent disagreement in the literature with respect to the definition of futility.

The Issue of Futility

While caring for terminally ill patients, physicians might be confronted with the question of whether to continue a therapy which they consider futile. The Task Force on Ethics of the Society of Critical Care Medicine pointed out that a healthcare professional has no obligation to offer, begin, or maintain a treatment which, in his or her best judgment, will be physiologically futile [4]. Nevertheless, caregivers should not assume that they understand the goals that a patient or family wish to achieve. Thus, caregivers should explicitly discuss goals and treatments to ascertain whether or not a treatment is of any value to the patient and family before determining that a treatment is inappropriate or inadvisable. For example, treatments that prolong the time until death may be viewed by some as useless or even harmful, because the treatments prolong dying or suffering. For others, these treatments may be considered valuable, since they permit the chance to share the experience of death with family members, provide an unlikely, yet desired, chance of survival, or are consonant with religious belief. In addition, some patients may want to undergo a treatment with a very low likelihood of success, particularly if it is their only chance for survival. These conflicts are typically about differences in values rather than disagreements about facts. In some circumstances, patients and families will request or even insist upon care that is not appropriate [8]. We have to remember that any treatment derives its medical justification from the benefits that the informed patient hopes to achieve by employing it [4].

The Principle of Beneficence

The principle of beneficence simply means the principle of doing good: what is the good that ought to be done? In medicine, beneficence means acting for the patient's benefit and for the promotion of his health and recovery: *bonum facere* or *salus aegroti suprema lex*. The principle of beneficence encompasses the fundamental goals of medicine which are [6]:
- The preservation of life
- The restoration of health
- The relief of suffering
- The restoration or maintenance of function

These are all positive steps and these values should guide medical treatment. However, the question remains: How to know what is good and what is harmful? The politically correct answer is simple: ask the patient. Because of the divergent understandings of what should count as actually "doing good", Engelhardt [2] points out that one cannot understand (in tems of secular morality) the principle of beneficence simply as the Golden Rule. If one does unto others as one would have them do unto oneself, one may in fact be imposing on others against their will a particular view of the good life [2]. The Golden Rule can thus be the basis for the paternalistic imposition of particular understandings of the "good life". To avoid such paternalism, Engelhardt [2] phrases the principle of beneficence in the positive form: "Do to others their good." However, any talk of the best interests of others presupposes a particular judgment about what constitutes those best interests. When one speaks across moral communities, different judges of best interests with different moral senses are presupposed. The maxim "Do to others their good" must be understood as "Do to others their good, unless one recognizes the purported good to be harm or the provision of the good to be in some sense wrong" [2]. Because of conflicts among the diverse visions of the good, the good one recognizes that one ought to do to others will frequently be seen by those others as harm. One may then be forbidden by the principle of respect for autonomy to do to others what one sees to be their good, but which they regard as harmful. The morality of mutual respect gives to individuals the right to veto the provision of a good they do not want. On the other hand, the moral insights of one's own moral background may forbid doing to others what they hold to be good but which one knows to be evil or harmful.

To summarize this aspect: the benefit of a treatment depends on the physiologic outcome of the intervention, the probability of that outcome and the patient's perception of the benefit of that outcome [7]. Therefore, in case of conflict, we have to ask the patient.

The Principle of Nonmaleficence

The principle of nonmaleficence means that one ought not to inflict evil or harm: above all do not harm, or *primum non nocere* ! Nonmaleficence stands for avoiding anything that might have negative consequences, whereas beneficence means performing positive acts to promote good [1].

The Hippocratic oath, a guideline and recommendation for the medical professions in antiquity, combined the principles of nonmaleficence and beneficence: I will use treatment to help the sick according to my ability and judgment (which reflects the principle of beneficence), but I will never use it to injure or wrong them (which means nonmaleficence) [1]. For Engelhardt [2], nonmaleficence just means special application of the principle of beneficence. The principle of nonmaleficence underscores the fact that one will not be obliged to provide to others a service one finds to be a violation of the principle of beneficence. An individual might not object or, presumably, might consent to a harm, e.g., committing suicide, or the individual might not be able to refuse harm, due to a reduced consciousness or competence. Again, however, we are faced with the conflict that different views may exist of whether or not a treatment represents harm.

The Principle of Justice

The principle of justice affects priorities in the allocation of health care resources. Justice may be defined as giving to each person that which is due or owed and which can be legitimately claimed. It is a matter of justice to ensure some degree of equitable distribution of medical resources to all citizens. For instance, performing CPR although it is inappropriate or futile might delay or prevent emergency treatment in other patients with a better chance of survival. As we all know, this conflict is not restricted to the application of CPR efforts or to the use of expensive and scarce resources, such as critical care beds. In times when the demands on the health care system are heavily competing due to cutbacks in governmental financial policy, it is increasingly important to provide distributive justice by common agreement.

Conclusion

Ethical decisions in terminal illness are generally made on an individual basis. On critical or palliative care units, an atmosphere of close clinical supervision is usually found. Treatment decisions can be communicated to the relatives, to all members of the health care team, and sometimes to the patient. Ethical conflicts in terminal illness are difficult to resolve. The way they are solved by health care professionals is influenced by a wide variety of personal beliefs and religious and cultural differences. Ethical guidelines are needed since we all are facing moral pluralism. Moral diversity is real, and health care policy must be framed within this moral chaos. Ethical principles should serve as a supportive instrument in decision making. A sound ethical analysis of the specific case, based on the knowledge of the relevant principles – respect for autonomy, beneficence, nonmaleficence, and justice – will help to make a decision meeting the values and the interests of the patient. In conflicts, ethics committees could be helpful in decision making. However, in individual cases, ethical questions and conflicts without clear solutions may still remain.

References

1. Beauchamp TL, Childress JF (1994) Principles of biomedical ethics, 4th ed. Oxford University Press, New York
2. Engelhardt HT Jr (1996) The foundations of bioethics, 2nd ed. Oxford University Press, New York
3. Murphy DJ, Burrows D, Santilli S et al (1994) The influence of the probability of survival on patients' preferences regarding cardiopulmonary resuscitation. N Engl J Med 330:545-549
4. Task Force on Ethics of the Society of Critical Care Medicine (1990) Consensus report on the ethics of foregoing life-sustaining treatments in the critically ill. Crit Care Med 18:1435-1439
5. Thomas PD, Runciman WB (1996) Ethical Issues. In: Johnston JR (ed) International handbook of Intensive Care. Euromed Communications, Belfast, pp 1-12
6. Snider GL (1991) The do-not-resuscitate order. Ethical and legal imperative or medical decision? Am Rev Respir Dis 143: 665-674
7. Crimmins TJ (1993) Ethical issues in adult resuscitation. Ann Emerg Med 22:495-501
8. The Ethics Committee of the Society of Critical Care Medicine (1997) Consensus statement of the Society of Critical Care Medicine's Ethics Committee regarding futile and other possibly inadvisable treatments. Crit Care Med 25:887-891

Main Symbols

AR	Androgen receptors
AMPA	Alpha-amino-3-hydroxy-5-methyl-4-isoxazoleproprionate
APN	Acute pain nurse
APS	Acute postoperative pain Services
ASICs	Acid-sensing ion channels
BK	Bradykinin
CGRP	Calcitonin gene-related peptide
ChAT	Cholineacetyltransferase
CNS	Central nervous system
CRT	Controlled randomised trial
DNIC	Diffuse noxious inhibitory control
DRG	Dorsal root ganglion
EA	Epidural analgesia
fMRI	Functional magnetic resonance imaging
GDX	Gonadectomized
5HT	Serotonin
H	Hystamine
IASP	International Association for the Study of Pain
IPSPs	Inhibitory postsynaptic potentials
LEPs	Laser-evoked potentials
M3G	Morphine-3-glucuronide
M6G	Morphine-6-glucuronide
MCS	Motor cortex stimulation
NGF	Nerve growth factor
NMDA	N-metyl-D-aspartame
NO	Nitric oxide
PCA	Patient-controlled analgesia
PET	Positron emission tomography
PGE$_2$	Prostaglandins
PSPs	Postsynaptic potentials
RA	Regional Anaesthesia
rCBF	Regional cerebral blood flow
RT	Reticularis thalamus
SCS	Stimulation for chronic pain
SCS	Spinal cord stimulation
SEPs	Somatosensory evoked potentials
SPET	Single photon emission tomography
SRD	Subnucleus reticularis dorsalis
SRTT	Spino reticulo thalamic tract
STT	Spino thalamic tract
TTX	Tetrodoxin
VAS	Visual analogic scales

Subject Index

Acute pain, 11, 38, 41, 51, 57, 87, 89, 91-98
Allodynia, 14, 15, 17, 23, 26, 82, 85, 86
Anaesthesia, 17, 76, 96, 97, 99, 101, 103, 104
Analgesia, 9, 11, 12, 16, 17, 22, 25, 57, 72, 79, 81, 84, 86-94, 96-101, 104, 107-109
Autopoiesis, 55, 56, 58
Axonal injury, 15

Bradykinin, 11-13, 20, 22, 24
Brain, 5, 12, 16, 17, 25-27, 33-36, 42, 45, 48, 49, 51-58, 61, 64, 68, 70, 71, 73, 79, 82-87, 96
Brainstem reticular, 27

Cancer, 41, 57, 96-98, 104-110
Capsaicin, 12, 17, 21, 22, 25
Caudal brainstem, 27
Cholecystokinin, 12, 15, 24
Consciousness, 33, 38, 51, 52, 54-58, 114, 117
Corticotropin, 22

Dorsal root ganglia, 10, 13, 16, 18, 22, 61
Dysesthesia, 23

Electrophysiological assessment, 71, 84
Endorphin, 48
Ethical
 decision, 111, 117
 theories, 111, 112
Fast track, 99, 100, 103
Fentanyl, 57, 86, 109
Formalin test, 17, 43-47, 49

Galanin, 16, 18, 24
Glutamate, 9, 11-13, 88, 96

Hyperalgesia, 13-15, 17, 20, 21, 23, 24, 26, 62-70, 85, 106
Hyperpathia, 23, 41, 82

Inflammation, 10, 13-15, 17, 20-22, 24, 25, 60, 63, 66, 69
Informed consent, 113
Injury, 9, 13-18, 20, 22-24, 26, 39-42, 51, 53, 63, 66, 75, 76, 97, 101
Interleukin 1 beta, 22

Judgements, 111, 112, 115-117

Limbic brain, 53
Lymphocytes, 11, 22

Macrophages, 11, 22
Mediators, 20-23, 60
Methadone, 109
Monocytes, 11, 22
Morphine, 11, 16, 57, 80, 96, 97, 104, 106-110

Naloxone, 53, 43-46, 48, 72
Nerve growth factor, 9, 17, 18, 49
Nerve injury, 13, 15, 23, 24, 26, 42
Neurochemical substrate, 9, 12
Neurochemistry, 2, 9, 10
Neuromodulation, 71, 73, 74
Neuron, 4-11, 14-26, 34, 35, 37-40, 42, 43, 47-49, 55, 61, 64-66, 69, 80, 81, 83, 85, 86
Neuroscience, 1, 2, 4, 6, 7, 18, 34-36, 48, 96
Nitric oxide, 9, 17, 18

Subject Index

Nociception, 13, 17, 22, 32, 33, 37, 42, 51, 57, 59, 60, 68, 79, 84, 87
Nociceptive neurons, 10, 21, 80, 81
Nociceptors, 11, 12, 16, 19-26, 30, 55, 60, 65, 66, 69, 87, 96

Opioids, 12, 16, 22, 48, 49, 87, 90, 91, 94, 105-110

Pain, 9-20, 2, 23, 25-28, 30-43, 48, 49, 51-60, 62-65, 67-103, 105-110, 115
    control, 71, 75, 78, 80, 83, 84, 92, 105
    perception, 9, 12, 14, 53, 57
Paraesthesia, 23, 74
PET-scan, 71, 73, 80, 84
Postoperative analgesia, 91, 93, 96, 101

Regional anaesthesia, 17, 90, 91, 96, 97, 99, 104

Schwann cells, 15, 18
Sensory neurons, 10, 11, 13-19, 21, 23, 24, 39, 64

Somatic pain, 59, 64
Spinal cord, 10, 12-18, 24, 28, 30, 32-35, 37-39, 42, 51, 53, 54, 61, 64, 71, 73, 74, 77, 83-89, 96, 101
Spinal pathways, 27, 28, 39
Sufentanil, 108, 109
Substance P, 10-12, 20, 21, 23, 88, 96
Surgery, 2, 44, 51, 57, 83, 85, 87-89, 93-97, 99, 100, 103, 104, 107

Terminal illness, 105, 111-113, 117
Testosterone, 43, 45-49
Thalamus, 30-33, 35, 37-42, 53, 61, 79-82, 86

Ventilatory support, 111
Visceral
    nociception, 59, 60, 68
    pain, 59, 60, 62, 64, 67-70
    sensitivity, 60

Wallenberg's syndrome, 30, 80
World Health Organization, 105

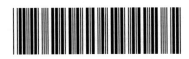